Prevent Cancer

AND A WHOLE LOT MORE

Nick Pagliarulo

Battle Press
SATELLITE BEACH, FLORIDA

Prevent Cancer
And A Whole Lot More

Battle Press books may be ordered through booksellers or by contacting:

Battle Press
1-919-218-4039
steve@battlepress.media

ISBN: 978-1-5136-7116-1 (softcover)
ISBN: 978-1-5136-7118-5 (eBook)

Library of Congress Control Number: 2021904859

First Edition

Table of Contents

Dedication

This book is dedicated to all those who lost loved ones to Cancer.

Thanks

Giving Thanks to my wonderful wife Nanet who assisted me in so many ways and allowed me to have the time needed to complete this book.

I would also like to express my gratitude to the many people who have seen me through the writing of this book by providing support, exploring ideas, offering constructive comments, and assisting in the editing and proofreading process.

Foreword

Hello to all. I am a 58 year old Paramedic licensed in the state of Florida. I worked on an ambulance as the lead paramedic for over 25 years, responding to 911 calls for people in need of medical attention from traumatic injuries to medical emergencies. I accomplished and performed pretty much every possible procedure that there is to do, including lifesaving, cricothyrotomies, pleural needle decompressions, synchronized and unsynchronized cardioversions and endotracheal intubations. I worked an overwhelming amount of overtime and was able to see a wide variety of acute medical emergencies and chronic medical conditions.

I always paid attention to my patient's complaints and treated them accordingly, but it was not until I started this wonderful, clean living journey did I start to realize that the majority of these patients' medical conditions were because of their diet and/or living conditions. Prime examples are diabetic patients with soda cans and candy wrappers throughout the house, or asthma or COPD patients living with multiple pets with a carpeted home collecting dust and dander. Or the Asthma patient spraying air fresheners throughout the house.

This is when I noticed that these patients are living in a vicious cycle that probably will never change unless they make changes in their diet and lifestyle. Without knocking our healthcare system, there are not a lot of proactive preventive treatments. They do, however, provide a pamphlet upon discharge that is filled with good information, but unfortunately the majority of these are thrown away. It would be great if there was follow up care regarding some suggested lifestyle changes, especially for our chronic hospital patients.

Unfortunately, our healthcare system consists of treating you with medications which have a multitude of side effects that can cause their own medical conditions, instead of preventive medicine which could keep you home and healthy.

For the last eight years I currently own and operate a bread route in one of our major supermarkets. This is where I was able to see a large number of shopping carts filled with products that are unhealthy. So many people are buying a multitude of products that are simply not good for them. Everything I've learned through my careers is what inspired me to write this book, as I want to bring to light many unhealthy ingredients that are probably causing you and your family medical ailments, up to and including Cancer.

Join me on this journey and allow me to be your health and nutrition coach. I will continue to inform you of healthy choices to keep you and your family healthier and Cancer free.

Subscribe to my YouTube Channel:

Clean Living Club With Nicky P:
https://www.youtube.com/channel/UCd4mH8mA4Y8rtXK1_RHC09Q

Enjoy,

Nick Pagliarulo

Introduction

I wrote this book to help people as I have done my entire career in EMS, but in a different way. My objective is to teach you simple steps so you can use common sense decision making to protect you and your family from Cancer, viruses and a multitude of medical conditions. I am sure you are familiar with many of the recommendations that I am about to present to you, but I will simplify many things so you can begin a gradual, life-long journey of living a cleaner and healthier life.

In this book you will not only learn simple ways to eat healthy but ways to keep your house and surroundings safer. There are so many harmful products that we use on an everyday basis that I feel are not only a waste of money, but a key factor in weakening your immune system.

There are hundreds of health books and videos out there with a lot of great information. In this short book I will cut to the chase and tell you several ideas that I think you should try to implement in your life, and others you should eliminate. If you do, I promise you, you will not only look and feel healthier but your immune system will be stronger than ever. You probably will not have the everyday ailments like headaches, sinus problems, fatigue, and skin irritabilities and a list of others, these will become a thing in the past. The majority of these everyday illnesses are self-induced and easily preventable, as you will learn in this book.

There are some known facts of harmful chemicals that are in many of the products we use every day. Unfortunately no one is bringing it to our attention, instead they are trying to

---

sell us more of it. For instance, our women of the world are using a multitude of hygiene products that contain harmful chemicals that are known as Carcinogens.

In this book I will be the one to get on a soapbox and bring to your attention many of the harmful chemicals that we use in hopes that you make subtle changes in your life and discontinue their use.

This book contains:

- An 18 step guide to build your immune system (pages 23-24).
- A list of The Dirty Dozen fruits and vegetables to avoid unless buying organic (page 76).
- A list of the Clean 15 fruits and vegetables you should eat (page 77).
- A list of 50 Big Switches you should try to implement in your life (pages 83-85).
- The difference between processed and highly processed foods and what you should know (Chapter 9).
- A list of toxic ingredients in your household and hygiene products that you should avoid (Chapter 4).

As you digest all of this information, I know it will be hard to adhere to all of the suggestions, but keep them in mind because they are in you and your family's best interest. Use this book as a reference as you continue to walk the path of a healthier life.

Chapter 1
What is Causing all the Cancer?

The main objective of this book is to bring to your attention the many ingredients and harmful chemicals that might be causing you and your loved ones illnesses, and to aid you in preventing Cancer. In order to accomplish these goals we must take immediate action to build your immune system and not tear it down.

I am not going to go into full detail in this chapter of all the chemicals we come into contact with, and the carcinogens that we actually put in or on our bodies. I want to use this chapter as a lead in as what is to come. I want to feed you full of great information that will strengthen your family's immune systems and help combat the risk of Cancer.

I hope I will earn your trust as I have nothing to gain by giving you false information. No one is paying me to warn you of our common household Cancer causing environments that we create without realizing it. No one else is telling you that many of our common illnesses very well could be from our food source and our self-created toxic environment. I want to bring to light some basic everyday items like air fresheners that could be causing you terrible headaches and lead to more serious conditions, up to and including Cancer.

With that said, there are only 4 major routes by which carcinogens may enter your body:

1. Inhalation through the nose and mouth (this is most common).
2. Absorption through the skin and eyes.
3. Ingestion through swallowing.
4. Injection through needles and puncture wounds.

These chemicals go from the lungs and skin directly into the bloodstream. It is my goal that you realize how easy it is to poison yourself, and how these chemicals and carcinogens could be causing your headaches, fatigue, skin rashes and other ailments that may be early indicators of what could develop into Cancer.

We still don't know and probably never will know exactly what is causing all the Cancer. We do know that carcinogens entering your body is a high probability of what is causing the Cancer.

What Is Cancer?

Cancer is defined as a group of diseases involving abnormal cell growth with the potential to invade or spread to other parts of the body. There are over 100 types of Cancer affecting humans. Common symptoms include a lump, abnormal bleeding, prolonged cough, unexplained weight loss, and a change in bowel movements.

Make Note

Bowel movements are not mentioned again in this book so please make note that any change or abnormality in your stool seek medical attention immediately. Don't wait.

The Risk Factors of Cancer include:

- Obesity
- Tobacco
- Poor diet
- Lack of physical activity
- Excessive alcohol
- Certain infections
- Hazardous environment

In this book I will key in on only a few risk factors. We all know tobacco and alcohol can lead to Cancer. In this book I want to emphasize on a poor diet, obesity, and your living environment and hope to bring to light how these factors are becoming more harmful as our food is filled with toxic chemicals.

Newsflash

Obesity is now the number one cause of preventable death in the U.S. according to research presented at the 2017 Society of General Internal Medicine Annual Meeting.[1] Tobacco use was at the top of the list for decades, but as more and more people

---

[1] Obesity is top cause of preventable life-years lost, Science Daily, Apr 22, 2017, https://www.sciencedaily.com/releases/2017/04/170422101614.htm

have stopped smoking, with more and more people eating un-healthy foods, obesity is now the number one cause. Obesity is also one of the main risk factors of many Cancers. It is time that we as a whole realize that obesity from a poor diet is tak-ing more lives than smoking.

Feeding of the Masses

The more I have researched, the more I have come to the conclusion that eating and living like the vast majority of peo-ple (what I call "feeding of the masses") will lead to an un-healthy lifestyle and a weak immune system. This is opening the door for medical conditions like viruses and eventually possibly Cancer invading your body. Removing yourself from the feeding of the masses is essential. This is where you need to step outside the box and guide you and your family to a healthier lifestyle. Being mindful of what touches or enters your body through ingestion, inhalation, absorption and injection will produce a healthier life with less ailments, medications, and of course doctor visits.

Buying organic products and eating grass fed beef is a huge start and here I will briefly tell you why. This is a huge step to remove yourself from feeding of the masses. Yes, many of our organic foods are still processed but they do not contain the harmful toxic ingredients that I will mention in the upcoming chapters. Yes, Grass fed beef still comes from a slaughterhouse, and maybe the same one, but the cows are not pumped with hormones and antibiotics that are causing a multitude of medi-cal conditions, like obesity and diabetes, which are leading risk factors leading to Cancer.

In this book I hope to encourage you to eliminate your processed meats as they are proven to be harmful for you and that they can cause Cancer. There should be no mystery in the meat that you eat. Take the mystery out of the meat and keep it simple. Simple logical things, like eating ethically raised animals, and realizing that farm raised fish and shrimp contain chemicals that may also cause you and your family medical conditions, and are known to lead to Cancer. Most of your fast food, sushi bars and buffets all serve farm raised products that are unhealthy. They are giving you protein, and yes they provide you basic nutrients, but they are most likely causing you harm. Frequent long term ingestion of farm raised shrimp and fish are unhealthy and probably causing you or your family some type of medical condition.

Chapter 2
COVID-19
The Virus The Pandemic

How COVID-19 Inspired me Even More to Write this Book

When I started writing this book our current Pandemic was simply a strand of the Coronavirus. I am going to give you my non-political opinion as I bring to light our society's initial outlook about this virus. At first our leaders told us that the virus was not a threat to the United States and wearing a mask was not necessary. Things changed rapidly and drastically, and this highly contagious virus eventually infected millions of people as our country was under attack and still is.

Who Gets Sick

We have learned that healthy individuals infected by the Virus might not experience any signs or symptoms. We have also learned that unhealthy people that are infected may become gravely ill and possibly die. With the virus being highly contagious, this is why it became a Pandemic. If the majority of the people infected became ill, it would have been much easier to contain and it would most likely have been classified as a bad flu and certainly not be causing the massive hospitalizations and death toll that our country has endured.

A Healthy America Equals No Pandemic

So we know that this virus attacks and sickens individuals with a weak immune system. We also know that people with strong immune systems probably will not even know they have the virus. With this being said, you can see how a healthy diet and living clean can have a direct impact on our entire world health. If we absorb, inhale and ingest less chemicals in our bodies our immune systems will be so much stronger that not one virus could ever impact society.

Stay Healthy

This is why I encourage you to reduce you and your family's exposure to chemicals and to enhance your diet with great nutrients and real food, and less highly processed food additives (chemicals) in your diet.

Chapter 3
Build Your Immune System

Before I give you some great advice on building your immune system, I want to simply define our amazing fighting machine.

Our Amazing Fighting Machine

Our bodies house a dynamic natural-fighting machine, so intelligent and mighty. It does not rest and constantly fights. It allows you to come into contact with many harmful chemicals on a regular basis. It also allows you to contact a multitude of viruses and bacteria's without you even knowing it. Unfortunately, as we grow older and we continue to come in contact with carcinogens, our mighty immune system weakens; not because of age, as much, but because of the constant exposure of harmful chemicals. This allows Cancer and many other diseases to develop.

What is Your Immune System?

Your immune system is a complex network of mighty cells and proteins that defend the body against infection and illness. It is more sophisticated than the smartest computer as it keeps a record of every germ/microbe it ever defeated so it can always recognize it and defeat it again.

The immune system consists of white blood cells searching for foreign invaders. When invaders are detected the immune system sends B cells, T cells, and other killer cells to fight the intruder antibodies. The white cells fight toxins in your body as well as toxins you come into contact with through touch.

There are four parts of the immune system:

1. **The Complement System** is made up of strong proteins which aid the antibodies.

2. **The Lymphatic System** deals with Cancer cells early. Lymphatic cells also react to bacteria and deal with the dying cells that could turn into Cancer or other diseases.

3. **The Thymus** filters your blood and produces white blood cells.

4. **Bone marrow** is a spongy tissue inside your bones that creates red blood cells.

These are the components of the immune system that actively fight infection. It is amazing how many viruses and bugs your body battles on a daily basis. If you get sick a lot, including the common colds, there is a good chance your immune system could be a lot stronger.

Most people with strong undamaged immune systems rarely get sick. In fact there are documented cases where people have successfully combated Cancer through the means of only boosting their immune system to treat Cancer.

In my opinion, without a doubt keeping the immune system strong is the most important thing that can be done for your health. Being healthy on the inside is much more important than looking healthy on the outside.

Follow this Program to Build Your Immune System

1. Men, drink a gallon of filtered water a day (chemical free). Women should drink three-quarters of a gallon. Proper hydration removes toxins and has many other positive functions I will discuss later in the book.
2. Take a quality probiotic. I am not big on a lot of capsules and pills but this one is essential.
3. Get seven or eight hours of quality sleep a night.
4. Avoid added sugars.
5. Eat more whole plant veggies, nuts and seeds.
6. Add healthy fats like olive oil and coconut oil. They do not have to be organic.
7. Be active in activities such as walking, working out, or basic exercising.
8. Reduce stress.
9. Take naps, meditate or pray.
10. Consume garlic.
11. Drink organic green tea.
12. Take organic green leaf powder supplement several times a week. Mix it with organic beet powder.
13. Drink another half a gallon of filtered water if you are working out or profusely sweating.
14. Consume Prebiotics. Prebiotics feed your probiotic. Examples of Prebiotic foods are apple cider vinegar (ACV), tomatoes, asparagus, bananas, onions, garlic and whole oats.
15. Add Cilantro to your diet as it enhances excretion of lead and other heavy metals.

16. Consume good quality protein like organic eggs, organic beef and almonds.
17. ACV/ Apple Cider Vinegar (make sure it says "With the Mother").
18. Herbs: I encourage you to expand your journey and look into all the powerful herbs and implement them in your diet. My top 3 herbs are ginger, cilantro and turmeric as they contain a multitude of antioxidants and Cancer fighting ingredients. I call them my 3 superheroes. Put these superheroes in your diet today.

As I began following these steps I felt a mental and physical connection as my brain started to communicate with my body. Start following these steps and you will change from the inside and your desire for junk food will fade away. And when you do slip, there will be a mental reaction and your brain will trigger thoughts immediately like "Why did I eat that?"

Building your immune system not only aids in preventing Cancer, but your colds and viruses will be fewer and farther between, and could keep you from ever getting sick again.

Keeping your immune system strong is the most important thing you can do for yourself and your family. The physical fitness part will come later. Your healthy journey begins with getting your insides in shape. As a nutrition coach, I can help you do this in no time. Follow the above steps as your guide. Once you start this process and consume the above nutrients you and your family will feel and look healthier.

Drink Clean Water

Buy a quality filtration system for your home or just buy a few pitchers and remove the harmful chemicals in your water.

This is one of my strongest recommendations. You need to drink a lot of water and it needs to be good water. There is a lot more in upcoming chapters about water.

Chapter 4
Beware of Carcinogens!

A carcinogen is a substance capable of causing Cancer to a living tissue.

Are You Damaging You and Your Family's Immune System?

My goal in this chapter is to bring to light and inform you of some of the hideous chemicals you and your family are being exposed to. We all take for granted these popular products that make our hair and skin shine are healthy. And we think because our clothes are so white and clean that we should be grateful we can afford such wonderful products. And we are safe because we clean with this expensive disinfectant that kills 99% of all germs. However, many of the products we use every day are made up of toxic chemicals that enter your bloodstream through absorption and inhalation.

Why are Carcinogens Allowed in the Products you put in Your Body?

I cannot, for the life of me, even answer that question. Once I started this journey, I quickly realized that our society's problem is not just the chemicals we like to consume in our diet, but equally disturbing is the hideous chemicals we absorb through our skin, which includes nails and hair. Because you are not ingesting these chemicals, somehow our world governments feel its ok for you to wash your child's hair with known carcinogens. It's ok to scrape carcinogens with a stainless-steel blade into your skin. So of course, it's ok to wash our clothes with toxic chemicals and known carcinogens. Remember that if it is capable of causing Cancer, it can cause many other medical conditions. Can these chemicals cause migraines, vertigo, fatigue, depression and skin rashes? Well of course they can!

Build Your Immune System by not Weakening It!

The best thing you can do for your immune system is to not damage it. Again, so many products we use like soaps, shampoos, lotions, deodorants and cleaners are doing you and your family harm. Our women's feminine hygiene products have Cancer causing chemicals that are also hormone disruptors. In most cases these chemicals do not immediately cause medical conditions. This makes it difficult post-chemical consumption for your doctor to diagnose you properly because he or she has no idea what chemicals you put in or on your body every day. Your doctor can diagnose you with migraines, but he can only guess why you are getting them— and it sure is not going to be because you are using a lot of household chemicals or hair dies. He may get close every now and then and ask you if you are using any new detergents or soaps, but he is still so far off. Just because you stop using one chemical, it does not mean the 100 other chemicals are not causing you harm. Chances are you might be diagnosed with an allergic reaction to a new soap or detergent if they dug that deep with questioning, depending on your complaint.

Unfortunately, our healthcare system is not designed to diagnose a slow reaction to chemicals that are used every day. They are so subtle and affect different people in different ways, and some people are not affected at all. It is my belief these chemicals we use every day are slowly tearing down your immune system. I hope someday the medical community will look more in depth as to why so many patients have weak immune systems. I hope they take into consideration that our supermarket shelves are filled with a lot of harmful chemicals. It is my belief that these everyday chemicals we come into contact with are causing most of the Cancers.

Let's Talk Chemicals

Ladies first. I find this alarming and you should as well. Some of our feminine hygiene products contain a well-known carcinogen called Paraben.[2] Paraben is an active ingredient in vaginal creams and several other creams and lotions. Not only is it a carcinogen, it is being deemed more potent than they thought. Paraben increases breast cell growth and is linked to breast Cancer. Yes, you can still buy these products today.

Another chemical linked to breast Cancer is Phthalates.[3] Phthalates are found in panty liners and feminine pads. Ladies use caution here. Phthalates are also found in hairspray, nail polish, soaps and shampoos. They are also found in lotions, perfumes and more. Most perfumes on the market are toxic and unhealthy causing headaches and skin abnormalities and should be labeled as such. This is why I say step outside the box and start using organic and natural products. Essential

[2] Exposure to Chemicals in Cosmetics, Breastcancer.org, https://www.breast-cancer.org/risk/factors/cosmetics
[3] Phthalates, Breast Cancer Prevention Partners, https://www.bcpp.org/resource/phthalates/

oils are a great alternative for you and they smell amazing. Find good reputable companies that make quality products.

Phthalates are also linked to:

- Obesity
- Asthma
- Decreased fertility
- Hormone disruption
- Developmental issues

More Personal Products

Sodium Laureth Ether Sulfate (SLES) is an accepted chemical that is very inexpensive and a very effective foaming agent that is in most toothpastes, soaps, shampoos, shaving creams and many more. Although there is no direct link to Cancer it is being studied and on many Cancer watchdog lists. However, it is known to cause the following medical conditions and complaints:

- Hormonal disruptions
- Headaches
- Skin rashes
- Dermatitis
- Eczema
- Eye irritation
- Psoriasis

How many of us are going to the doctor and being given some medication to treat the above symptoms?

Let's Wash Some Clothes

I hate to continue to be the bearer of bad news, but it is in your and your family's best interests. One of our leading laundry detergents (and many others) contains another hideous chemical that is classified as a carcinogen. Dioxane is considered a carcinogen by the Environmental Protection Agency (EPA).[4] They state that short term inhalation to exposure of high levels of Dioxane causes several ailments such as:

- Headaches
- Skin irritation
- Dizziness

These carcinogens smell really good and many commercials advertise the fresh clean scent will last for days. Well here's another newsflash: It's not fresh. It's a poison that will make you sick and might even give you Cancer. Doesn't that make you want to take a big whiff of that clean towel? I highly recommend safer laundry detergents. If you do continue to use these best sellers please try to avoid any contact with the liquid or powder and don't over-do-it with the quantity you pour in and of course wash with the extra rinse cycle.

Are We Washing Our Hair With Carcinogens?

The answer is yes. According to several studies on soaps and shampoos, the products you use to wash your hair may cause Cancer. There are hundreds of chemicals in shampoos,

---

[4] The Hidden Carcinogen in Laundry Detergents and Bubble Bath: 1,4 Dioxane, https://littleloveorganics.com/blogs/news/the-hidden-carcinogen-in-laundry-detergents-and-bubble-bath-1-4-dioxane

and I find it quite disturbing. So many have been linked to Cancer, but apparently that is not proof that it causes Cancer. I recommend you check your shampoo labels for ingredients and avoid the product if it contains any of the following:

1. Sodium Lauryl Sulphate (SLS)
2. Fragrance
3. Cocamidopropyl Betaine
4. Triclosan
5. Polysorbates
6. Polyethylene Glycol (PEG)
7. Potassium Sorbate
8. PhenoxyEthanol
9. Retinyl Palmitate
10. Dimethicone
11. Behentrimonium Chloride
12. Quaternium-15

I also recommend using organic shampoos or keep it simple by using shea butter or a neem based soap. Again, we do not know what's causing all the Cancer. Maybe these chemicals won't cause you Cancer but maybe they will cause your family member Cancer. Maybe they will just cause headaches and dizziness. We will never know what's causing any medical complaint until we eliminate the possibilities. Be safe!

Air Fresheners

Air fresheners are one of our country's favorite toxic household products. There are a multitude of unwanted chemicals in most of these products and using a search engine you will find out that our country's leading products are on a list of toxic air fresheners. I will only mention one, and it is in most of the air fresheners.

Acetaldehyde is known to cause Cancer. Acetaldehyde also is a neurotoxin and immunotoxin—a known endocrine disruptor. 'Ace' is also known to cause skin, eye and lung irritability.[5]

Remember this: air fresheners do not eliminate the odor. They only mask the odor with a beret of toxic chemicals that are not only linked to Cancer but also to a host of medical complaints. Air fresheners are a main culprit of migraine headaches or headaches in general. If you have chronic headaches, pay attention to the use of air fresheners. Even the ones hanging in your car just above your nose. I encourage you to use essential oils as they are a great alternative and they smell amazing. Using distilled vinegar and water make a great car vinyl cleaner and you can also spray it on carpets without staining it.

Oven Cleaners and All Other Cleaners

Remember that there are a lot of harmful chemicals in cleaning products and the labels clearly say for you to not let it touch your skin. My personal opinion is that we waste a lot of money on these products that very well could be causing you and your family harm. We do not need to kill 99% of germs. Our Immune system will take care of it and actually makes it stronger. So killing every germ in your house is borderline absurd and actually harmful. You will be exposed to

---

[5] Toxic Chemicals in Air Fresheners, Madesafe.org, Jan. 19, 2020, https://www.madesafe.org/toxic-chemicals-in-air-fresheners/

these chemicals even if your maid is doing the cleaning. Remember, there is a chemical residue left all over your countertops or whatever was cleaned. In other words, you or your family are putting your hands on chemicals unless you rinsed with a freshly rinsed rag after cleaning. I am not sure how many housekeepers rinse their cleaned counter top. I am just giving you something to think about.

There are a lot of chemicals in these products, and I would use caution. Always wear a mask and gloves when cleaning and remember bleach is a known carcinogen. I personally use vinegar and water for basic cleaning. Bathrooms can be cleaned and effectively kill bacteria and viruses with water and only 10% bleach. Wear gloves and a mask of course and turn on the fan. If you are cleaning in a confined space with cleaning products, remember to have good cross ventilation even if you must bring in a fan. The fumes from many of these products are toxic and can cause you harm.

What about the Bug Man?

I am not even going to list the names of the chemicals in bug spray. There have been a lot of studies on bug repellants, but common sense should tell you they are not good for you. I don't want to put the bug man out of business, but I think you should know my personal opinion. These poisons will make you very sick. With that said, I am going to suggest to you a way to eliminate the need for any insect repellant. Stop feeding the bugs. Stop inviting them into your home. They are only doing what is natural. They are hungry.

Follow these quick steps and you will not need to pay a bug man or waste money on bug sprays:

1. Put all meat or sugary food wrappers in a box in the freezer or refrigerator until garbage day.
2. Do a quick rinse of your cans and bottles before putting them in your garbage.
3. Put your leftover scraps in the refrigerator – they are great for compost including eggshells.
4. Wipe down countertops with distilled vinegar and water regularly.

It does take a little time and a little labor but consider that you are keeping your family safe and that you are saving money. We have a small box in the freezer for our produce clippings, eggshells and banana peels. Your plants will love you.

Yard Care

I encourage you to try and eliminate pesticides and herbicides that are in your fertilizer. I understand most people will not adhere to this but at least keep it in mind and remember that those chemicals in your freshly sprayed yard are Carcinogenic and can cause you and your loved ones to get sick. I definitely would not wear the shoes that just walked on your chemically sprayed lawn in your home. Also the run-off of these chemicals from our yards into the streets can flow into bodies of water, polluting the water for generations to come.

Do You Live Near a Golf Course? FYI

If you do, definitely invest in a water filtration system. A proportionate mortality study of golf course superintendents found elevated levels of Cancer and neurological disease compared to the general public.[6]

A Few More Harmful Carcinogens Close To Home

The following are only two of the manufactured chemicals we created to put into products worldwide since the 1940s. They are known as Carcinogens. They are alarming and you need to be aware of their harmful effects.

- Perfluorooctanoic Acid (PFOA)[7]
- Per-and-Polyfluoroalkyl Substances (PFAS)[8]

We created these chemicals for a variety of industries and we have finally acknowledged they are causing illness up to and including Cancer. The Government is finally stepping up as the State of Florida Department of Health has put out a two page Chemical Awareness information warning listing the concerns and precautions one should take (See Appendix A).

---

[6] Health Effects – Golf – Perfect Earth Project, https://perfectearthproject.org/health-effects/golf

[7] Perfluorooctanoic Acid (PFOA), Teflon, and Releated Chemicals, American Cancer Society, https://www.cancer.org/cancer/cancer-causes/teflon-and-perfluorooctanoic-acid-pfoa.html#:~:text=IARC%20has%20classified%20PFOA%20as,limited%20evidence%20in%20lab%20animals.

[8] PFAS Chemical Awareness, Florida Department of Health, http://www.floridahealth.gov/environmental-health/hazardous-waste-sites/contaminant-facts/_documents/doh-pfas-poster.pdf

Unfortunately they are finding these chemicals in our beautiful bodies of water. The Government has also found these chemicals in drinking water. It is important to buy a good water filter.

PFAS are used to manufacture the following products (Buyer beware, read the labels):

- Stain resistant carpets (Go Tile).
- Waterproof mattresses and clothing!
- Grease resistant food packaging (Microwave popcorn bags, pizza boxes, baking paper, and lots of other food packaging).
- Printers and copy machines.
- Receipts! (Leave your receipt maybe? I do).
- Nonstick cookware and lots of other products.

The PFAS from these products are linked to:

- Cancer
- Liver disease
- Decreased fertility
- Asthma
- Thyroid disease

So chances are we come into contact with these carcinogens every day. The sad thing is like many poisons they are odorless and tasteless.

I encourage you to stay informed and join me on my upcoming YouTube channel and I will provide you useful information on these and other chemicals to keep you and your family safe.

Clean Living Club With Nicky P:
https://www.youtube.com/chan-
nel/UCd4mH8mA4Y8rtXK1_RHC09Q

Summary

We still do not know what's causing so many people to get Cancer. We can only assume the possibilities and prevent Cancer by eliminating the high probabilities. I am giving you my opinion as to what I believe will keep you and your family safe. I also strongly believe without a shadow of a doubt that some of the products you use every day cause Cancer and at the least wear down your immune system. Again, it's documented that these products contain carcinogens but we still do not think twice about using them. I encourage you to start to think twice and go one step further and start making changes. I also encourage you to do your own research and challenge my warnings.

The good news is there are a lot of healthy alternatives out there. I strongly recommend you keep your family safe and go online and start ordering natural chemical free soaps, shampoos and lotions. These products are easy to get and are becoming more and more popular because of the fast speedy delivery. Look at the ingredients you are putting on you and your family's bodies and make a good decision and make these simple changes.

Chapter 5
Plastics Can Cause Cancer

This Chapter is going to focus on the need for us as a society to start moving away from plastics as far as food and beverage containers are concerned. Plastics should be holding hardware like nails and screws etc. As far as food and beverages go, I am not sure if anything good for you comes in plastic. Avoiding food and beverages that are packaged in plastic is a big step in the right direction to keeping your family healthier.

Plastic bottles have several carcinogenic chemicals that will break down and leech into your water beverage and it will be ingested—possibly causing Cancer.

Human Carcinogens

BPA (BISPHENOLA A) is a well-known chemical that is now labelled a HUMAN carcinogen.[9] Most carcinogens are confirmed through animal testing and not confirmed as a human carcinogen until there is not a shadow of a doubt that it causes people Cancer. BPA is still in many products we use daily. Just recently we have BPA-free products available. So should we feel better now that a lot of bottles and plastic containers are

[9] Bisphenol BPA should be classified as a carcinogen, Breast Cancer UK, https://www.breastcanceruk.org.uk/news/bisphenol-bpa-should-be-classified-as-a-carcinogen/#:~:text=A%20recently%20published%20re-view%20of,in%20in%20vivo%20mammalian%20models

BPA free? Maybe a little. Unfortunately, there are dozens of other similar chemicals that the EPA is just getting around to testing. Chances are they will also be labeled a carcinogen soon, BPA has a couple of siblings that strongly suggest they will be recognized carcinogens also: Bisphenol S and Bisphenol F. These siblings of BPA are already under heavy scrutiny along with a list of others. My point is, please, do yourself and your family a great big favor and start avoiding plastics and start using glass and stainless-steel containers. Use plastic containers to hold the nails and screws that you store in your shed, not your food. There are so many chemicals to talk about I just want to bring to light some of the chemicals that are known carcinogens and can and probably will cause you harm if you don't take a stand.

Ladies, BPA Causes Breast Cancer

It's in your feminine hygiene pads and several other hygiene products. BPA is in food containers, food cans, water supply lines, bottle tops, and of course plastic wrappers. I again ask you to start being mindful of any plastic. Try and start to eliminate it. Be mindful of your hygiene products including your toothbrush. I know it sounds impossible to eliminate. But just being mindful and paying attention to what goes on or in your body will reduce your chances of getting Cancer. Again, please remember that BPA-free means nothing. There are so many other chemicals in plastic that are remarkably similar, and probably will be considered carcinogens in due time.

I encourage you all to do some research on heating plastics and especially overheating plastics. This is where a high content of carcinogens are produced and released into your food. Have you ever overheated your kids' TV dinner or mac and cheese? Maybe you overheated your food after a night out drinking. If so, you have opened Pandora's Box, and it's full of carcinogens. Microwave popcorn is one of the worst as far as BPA and phthalates leaching into your products. I also encourage you to avoid heating anything in plastic, even if it says microwave safe. It's only microwave safe if you do not overheat. Once you overheat, all bets are off, and you are poisoning yourself and your family. Even their own product label will warn you of that only because the FDA forced them to. OK, so if I do not overheat, it's ok, then right? So, they say, yes, I say no. This is a definite buyer beware situation, so again I ask you to put some thought into your decision making. Do the manufacturers of the product care if I get Cancer? They are focused on making money now, not on the long term effect of your family's health.

Be Kind to Mother Earth

Last, but not least, these plastics that we buy are destroying ecosystems as they choke out coral reefs and poison our waters and the fish that we eat. Literally billions of pieces of plastic are smothering coral reefs today. Things are not getting any better, as most countries do not even regulate dumping; they use our oceans as a garbage depot. An entire book could be written on plastic pollutants, so I just want to ask all of you to do your part and do what you can to keep your family healthy by trying to limit your plastic use.

Chapter 6
Cooking To Fight Cancer

Cooking Creates Carcinogens

In this chapter I would like to address some concerns I have about cooking and bring to your attention some of the horrendous carcinogens that we create by using high heat. Yes, we create Cancer causing chemicals by practicing unsafe cooking habits. This seems to be a well-kept secret as you never hear any of our TV chefs mention this. Some of these chefs should think twice about making high heat cooking look so appetizing and fun. Many of us can't wait to get home and fire up the grill. Most of the commercials on TV show people grilling outside, and they have high flames with meat on the grill. This is so wrong and unhealthy because this causes Cancer. I can only hope that more studies are being conducted where oncologists are asking Cancer patients if they frequently grilled their meat on high heat. I can only imagine that many people say a few times a week or yes every weekend. How about you? Do you love to grill? High heat, big flames?

Grilling meat, fish or chicken with high heat causes 2 chemicals to form: Polycyclic Aromatic Hydrocarbons (PAHs)[10] and Heterocyclic Amines (HCAs)[11]. They are both well known to cause Cancer in animals and highly suspected to increase the risk in humans.

Why isn't this Promoted?

We all love to watch cooking shows as many chefs teach you how to eat healthier. I have never once heard a chef inform us that high heat produces chemicals that may cause Cancer. Do you think you will ever see a commercial promoting Cancer prevention instead of Cancer treatment? I hope we do someday. One that starts off with a backyard BBQ with flames and meat cooking on the grill, and then showing Cancer patients being treated with their 10th chemo treatment laying on a stretcher with no hair.

With the commercial informing us of the carcinogens we create when cooking with high heat. Maybe we could get Cancer treatment centers to pay for commercials like these. Why would they do that? Prevention is not their game. There is simply no money in prevention. There are a dozen more scenarios of commercials that could inform us of the harmful things we do on a regular basis that may be causing you and your family harm. I find it saddening they do not inform us.

[10] Polycyclic Aromatic Hyrdocarbons: From Metabolism to Lung Cancer, Oxford Journals, May, 2015. https://www.ncbi.nlm.nih.gov/pmc/articles/PMC4408964/

[11] Chemicals in Meat Cooked at High Temperatures and Cancer Risk, National Cancer Institute, https://www.cancer.gov/about-cancer/causes-prevention/risk/diet/cooked-meats-fact-sheet

If you are grilling hotdogs on high heat, you are creating a lot of carcinogens as you cook. The hotdog alone can cause Cancer, but now we are releasing more chemicals using high heat.

Does anyone care why so many young people are getting Cancer? I do!

Many people do not know this, and again this is why I am writing this book. So let's use a common sense approach. I don't mean to rain on your backyard BBQ, I just want to inform you of a couple of possibilities that could be causing Cancer.

If you are going to grill I suggest the following:

1. Don't be in a rush.
2. Let your coals get gray before putting your meat chicken or poultry on the grill.
3. Cook on low heat. This goes for any cooking. I would not recommend charring any meat.
4. Cook slow and steady.
5. Never use the black coals, make sure they are gray. AVOID lighter fluid. It contains toxic hydrocarbons that are confirmed carcinogens. Chances are you are digesting this every time you grill if you use lighter fluid and black coals and high heat. Many skeptics will tell you that the fire burns off those chemicals.

Cook in Cast Iron and get Natural Supplemental Iron Intake

What we cook with is just as important as how we cook. For instance, did you know that cooking with cast iron actually gives you iron. Yes supplemental iron. Many women are deficient in this important mineral. It is clean and safe because you use low heat. Once your pans and pots are seasoned, cleanup is simple. They are heavy which can be cumbersome, so be careful! See Appendix A for instructions how to season and care for your cast iron pan.

A Little Aluminum or a Lot?

I would like to mention aluminum and talk about a few reasons not to use it when cooking.

Aluminum is found in a multitude of products, including water. We often get too much of it. This is my opinion again, but also many scientific studies cite there is a high possibility that aluminum toxicity is related to Alzheimer's, Parkinson's, and Cancer. So, when you are getting enough aluminum intake already, maybe it is a good idea not to get to the toxic level many scientists debate about.

As you start to walk this healthier living journey you will find the cleaner you eat, the less likely you will need an antiperspirant. The less chemicals you put into your body, the less body odor you will have. With that said, the aluminum in antiperspirants has been linked to breast Cancer.

If you still insist on cooking with aluminum again please never use high heat. This is when the aluminum and heat create carcinogens and are absorbed directly into your food. One of your favorite Italian restaurant chains uses high heat and Aluminum pans.

No Non-Stick Pans

There have been several studies and it is a known fact that for decades the chemical and carcinogen PFOA was found in non-stick pans. Only recently the manufactures have phased out this chemical because of its link to Cancer. They have stopped using the chemical only because of PFOA's negativity. Trust me, there are plenty more chemicals they are using to manufacture these non-stick pans that have not been studied yet. So I encourage you to keep your family safe and avoid nonstick pans.

Another Reason

As time goes on with everyday use or the pan is scraped with a sharp object these pans flake off material into your food. Now we have a foreign substance possibly lodged in your intestinal wall. I researched about these known potential flake offs and the search engine brought up articles advising me of good news. That digesting small flakes of nonstick coating is not dangerous. The material will most likely just pass through your body. And fortunately, MOST manufacturers of nonstick pans have phased out the use of Perfluorooctanoic Acid (PFOA), a suspected carcinogen.

I wanted to bring this to your attention as I found it disturbing that MOST manufacturers have stopped using PFOA's as an ingredient. Why not all? And having a piece of non-stick material being digested and hoping it just passes through. Or maybe it will be lodged in my intestines where a tumor might form. We must ask ourselves: "Why are so many people getting Cancer?"

My suggestion is to just skip the Cancer-causing pan and keep your family safe.

Beware of the Microwave

Caution: if you elect to use a microwave, never heat food in or on plastic. Not even microwave safe plates. Because once that microwave safe plate is overheated all bets are off. It is no longer safe and is actually releasing carcinogens'

They Say it is Safe

There have been a multitude off studies on microwaves and overwhelming studies state that microwaves are safe and they do not cause Cancer even if a person stands near it while it is in use. On the other hand if a pregnant woman stands too close to a leaking microwave it can be harmful. This is why they have the signs posted on the microwaves at convenience stores stating, "Microwave in use, if you are pregnant or have a pacemaker stand clear."

A microwave uses high frequency, high intensity signals that might interfere with a pacemaker.

Do they Leak Radiation?

Fact: If your microwave oven is broken, it can leak electromagnetic radiation. Microwave radiation leaks are extremely hard to detect because the radiation does not smell, and you cannot see it. So, you basically do not know if your microwave is leaking or how much it is leaking.

As I continued to do more research on microwaves I found out it is ok for a microwave to leak electromagnetic radiation. Low and behold, FDA regulations allow a small amount of leakage, about 5mW/cm2. But apparently we don't need to worry because the radiation is non-ionizing, so it will not damage your DNA directly, rather it will excite the water within your soft tissue. I am not sure about you but I will take a pass on my soft tissue getting excited, like that anyway.

Who Tests for Radiation Leakage?

I want you to pay close attention to this paragraph. Then you decide if it is safe for your family. The FDA allows manufacturers and businesses to sell you a new microwave that leaks a little bit of electromagnetic radiation. This is again disturbing. How old is the common household microwave? Google says 9-10 years (Digital Trends). How much electromagnetic radiation does an 8 year old microwave leak? As far as I know there is no one to call to see if your microwave is leaking. We are being told it is ok if a microwave leaks radiation and we can't monitor how much it is leaking. I only bring this information to you so you can make the decision on using microwaves. I wanted to bring to light some of the things no one tells us about.

Are Microwaves Causing Cancer?

Most studies say no they do not. I have no strong evidence that microwaves are causing Cancer. Microwaves became available for almost all households in the late 1970s. This is probably a big coincidence but Cancer cases exploded in the mid-1980s. Just a little food for thought.

Why are so many people getting Cancer?

Microwave Producing Carcinogens

Most of us live a busy life and microwaves are a part of many people's everyday lives. Just remember that when you are in a rush or come in from a night of drinking it is easy to overcook your food in a microwave. If you are overheating a microwave safe plate or a TV dinner in the microwave, you are without a doubt poisoning yourself with Cancer causing carcinogens.

More about Cooking

Perfluorooctanoic acid (PFC) is highly suspected to cause Cancer. This chemical is created when you have microwavable popcorn. If you overcook your microwavable popcorn, you have created several more chemicals that are carcinogens.[12] My opinion is that microwavable popcorn is very unhealthy without overcooking it. The bag alone contains unwanted chemicals.

---

[12] Microwave popcorn Causes Cancer: Fact or Fiction? Healthline, March 8, 2019, https://www.healthline.com/health/microwave-popcorn-cancer

Microwaves are your call. I have given my opinion. Remember they are allowed to leak radioactive rays and no one monitors it.

If you continue to use a microwave which most of you probably will, please avoid overheating plastic. I personally would not use any plastics in a microwave. Make sure your teenagers are aware of the Cancer it may cause as they often overcook the microwavable dinners. So protect your family and educate them on how to use the microwave as safe as they can.

Chapter Tips:

- Avoid aluminum pans and nonstick pans and use cast iron or stainless steel or glass.
- Don't overcook food in the microwave.
- Reconsider microwave use.
- Avoid using lighter fluid.
- Avoid high heat flames.
- Avoid black charcoal.

Chapter 7
Are You Drinking
Good Water?

Number 1 Recommendation: Drink a lot of Good Water

Let's make sure you are drinking enough good water. Men should intake close to 1 gallon of chemical-free water a day (of course more with profuse sweating). Women should drink about 3/4 of a gallon

We Need Water

We all know that drinking water is essential for you to maintain the balance of body fluids. It is also important to know that water is a major component in aiding your digestive system in removing toxins and carcinogens. It is probably the most important thing you can do for your health.

Your body is made up of 60% water. The function of these fluids is to aid in digestion, absorption and circulation, not to mention the transportation of your nutrients as well as helping to maintain a normal body temperature. Another important factor of water is the development of saliva which prevents gum disease, thrush and yeast infections in your mouth. Being dehydrated is the major cause for these illnesses of the mouth.

Drink Good Water

So we know that your body needs a lot of fluid intake to function properly. The more the merrier. If you drink a lot of water, and even if that's all you do at first, you are on the right track to a healthier lifestyle.

Urine

Urine is a key indication of your health. It is a way of your body letting you know if your fluid intake is good or bad. Your urine also will tell you if you are sick. Normally your urine should be a pale yellow, keeping in mind some foods and vitamins can change the color of your urine. Without getting too much in depth, please know that a deep amber is a sign of dehydration.

Foaming can simply be caused by the speed of your urination. Did you really have to go? In this situation you do not have anything to worry about. But if you have continuous foaming it could be an indication of a type of kidney failure and you should be evaluated by a doctor. Dark or orange urine is a probable sign of infection and it is time to see a Doctor. If you have any kind of pain while urinating also seek medical attention.

Fluid Options

There are so many beverages out there that claim to be good for you but in reality they are not. Granted, they might supply protein or caffeine and electrolytes which your body needs to function, but most of these drinks have an overabundance of sugar or artificial sweeteners that are unhealthy. Too much sugar is the sure path to diabetes and or obesity.

I can only tell you that if there is artificial flavor and colors in it, then it is not good for you. Many of us enjoy and want caffeine. Caffeine is not the problem. Rather, it is all the other added chemicals and sugars in these drinks that cause medical conditions including Cancer. High Fructose Corn Syrup (HFCS) is linked to Cancer and is a known cause of obesity, diabetes and heart disease to name a few.[13] I strongly recommend keeping it simple and just add good ingredients to your coffee, tea and water.

Option Drinks

Now that we are drinking clean, chemical free water, what about those drinks we discussed earlier in this chapter. I recommend that you try and put down the sugar and caffeine drinks as they will lead to medical complications and possibly Cancer. We do not know what's causing the Cancers.

Here are some suggestions I highly recommend. While getting your fluid intake you are getting great nutrients which is building your immune system.

- Add a few slices of lemon or lime in your water. They both have a multitude of nutritional benefits.

---

[13] High Fructose Corn Syrup: A Cancer Threat? Andrew Weil, M.D., Sept 27, 2010, https://www.drweil.com/health-wellness/body-mind-spirit/cancer/high-fructose-corn-syrup-a-cancer-threat/

- Add a splash of Apple Cider Vinegar (ACV). It is fresh and delicious, with or without lemon.
- Add a little ginger in your good water.
- Add a little turmeric in your good water.
- Drink Organic Green tea.
- Drink Organic coffee black.
- Stevia in my opinion is the way to go when you want a sweet drink. It is the healthier alternative.
- Raw Honey is good for you
- Organic beet powder
- Organic green vegetable powder

HAVE A DRINK ON ME!!

Chapter 8
Drinking Fluoride and Other Chemicals

I cannot emphasize the importance enough in this book of your water intake and your water being clean and chemical free. Because of my strong belief that our water could be causing Cancer and other diseases, I felt the need to do another chapter addressing fluoride and a few other chemicals that are used to treat water in most of our public water supply. After all, water is the main ingredient in staying healthy and building your immune system. We still do not know what's causing all the Cancer. Many of us think there is a strong correlation between the water we drink and Cancer. We can speculate and we can debate and there will always be strong points made on both sides. With that said, let's just keep things simple and clean as possible.

Do not Trust your City or County Water Supply

Get Your Water Tested!

I encourage you not to drink the water from your main water supply unless you personally have your water tested and researched to see what chemicals are in it. Think of it like reading the ingredients of a food label. If it is not good for you, do not consume it. Be mindful of washing your vegetables with your main water supply as these chemicals will remain on your food.

Water Filtration Systems

I know not everyone can afford a house filtration system as it might be in the area of $3000.00. Even a quality under the sink system will be about $300.00. A good quality pitcher that removes the fluoride costs about $40.00. I used the pitchers for years as they do a great job of removing harmful chemicals. It is a little cumbersome filling pitchers a few times a day, but quality water makes everything taste better and knowing you are keeping your family healthier is a giant step to living a cleaner life. I recommend a reverse osmosis system whether it be under the sink or a complete home system. Do your research and protect you and your family. Remember, it's not just Cancer we are trying to prevent. We are trying to prevent illness of any kind.

Ditch Bottled Water

I also strongly recommend that you and your family avoid bottled water or any beverage bottled in plastic, even if it is BPA FREE. The FDA allows bottled water companies to add a small amount of aluminum, nitrates and a few other unwanted chemicals. I find this absurd, but small amounts of these chemicals will not cause you harm we are told. The bottom line is that your beverage is housed in plastic that is made up of hundreds of chemicals. These chemicals can and will leach into your food or beverage. We have no idea how long that product was sitting in the sun or stored in a hot environment. When the plastic is heated it forms chemicals that are known carcinogens. There are so many unknowns when it comes to plastic bottles that we all just assume they are safe because they are for sale. I encourage you to make a stand

and dump the plastic as it is also a giant step on the road to clean living.

Unfortunately, bottled water is widely accepted and will most likely remain that way. How can we blame water bottles leaching chemicals as the reason your loved one got Cancer when it takes years of consuming these chemicals. We can't prove it so sadly plastic is here to stay. It is my opinion bottled water should be for natural disasters and not purchased for a convenient drink. The FDA does not regulate the amount of fluoride in bottled water. With that said, let's talk about fluoride again.

Fluoride

Fluoride is a natural-occurring mineral found in our natural waterways and is a natural chemical that is everywhere. This is not the problem. Unfortunately, synthetic fluoride is the culprit as far as I am concerned. Big companies and their lobbyists have succeeded in having synthetic fluoride added to our city and county water supply throughout the United States and the world. Using politics and convincing our local leaders the need for it to be added to the water because our children do not brush their teeth properly. That of course is my opinion on how it was implemented.

Fluoride and Cancer?

Although there is no direct evidence linking fluoride directly to Cancer, some studies have linked Fluoridation of water to have a detrimental effect on developing cells of the immune system and bone cells.[14] This could be a gateway for Cancer and at the least weaken your immune system allowing disease and sickness to invade your body. I mentioned this earlier but I feel it is important. I am not trying to convince you as much as I am wanting you to be educated and not to always trust what's being considered the normal. The normal almost seems to be getting Cancer and I know you don't want that. So again I encourage you to be the judge and do your own research and make your decision on what's safe for your family. Of course, there are plenty of articles warranting fluoride and reminding you that there is no concern of the levels you receive.

Skeletal Fluorosis

I believe you should be very concerned about too much Fluoride consumption as it is already in so many of the foods and beverages we ingest. Remember that it takes water to manufacture most of these foods and beverages and chances are the water probably contained fluoride. It is easy to see how we can accumulate too much fluoride and develop medical conditions like Skeletal Fluorosis. In many cases, Skeletal Fluorosis is misdiagnosed for many years or even decades as it mimics the chronic illness of arthritis.

---

[14] Effects of sodium fluoride on blood cellular immunity, Oncotarget, Aug 10, 2017, https://www.ncbi.nlm.nih.gov/pmc/articles/PMC5689626/

Below is a short list of products with high amounts of fluoride (Please make note that there are many more):

- Tea or coffee with tap water
- Fruit juices
- Sodas
- Canned Blue crab
- Canned Shrimp
- Wine
- Beer

In skeletal fluorosis, fluoride accumulates in the bones progressively over many years. It accumulates because of excess fluoride.[15] This causes bone pain and stiffness similar to arthritis which you may have been initially diagnosed with. Later, it progresses to crippling deformities of the spine and other joints. Canadian research studies have linked fluoride overexposure to ADHD and ADD. Other studies linked prenatal overexposure to fluoride to a lower IQ in children. The FDA has growing concerns and have urged bottled water companies to avoid adding fluoride to their products. With all this said, I again urge you to simply search the internet diligently and you will find these studies and statements from the FDA. You will also find articles that tell you that there is nothing to worry about. I ask you to be your own judge.

Waterborne Contaminants

Simply put, chlorine and chloramines need to be removed from your drinking water as they are known carcinogens.

---

[15] Fluoride in Drinking Water and Skeletal Fluorosis, Springer Link, Mar 23, 2020, https://link.springer.com/article/10.1007/s40572-020-00270-9

They are added to your tap water to kill bacteria. This is another big reason to buy a good water filter.

Below is a list of several other contaminants that should be removed and not consumed:

- Aluminum
- Ammonia
- Arsenic
- Barium
- Cadmium
- Chromium
- Copper
- Bacteria and Viruses
- Lead
- Nitrates
- Mercury
- Perchlorate
- Radium
- Selenium
- Silver
- Uranium

Many of the above contaminants are in your main water supply and are known carcinogens

More on Fluoride

I could write a small book on water fluoridation and may do so because of my stand against the added chemical. I will mention fluoride here again it is very important. I am giving you my opinion on what I strongly believe will keep your family safe. We don't know what's causing all the Cancer. Therefore, let's eliminate some strong possibilities.

I encourage you to take a stand on the fluoridation of water. Numerous studies have been done and some believe it was the greatest scientific mistake ever. With that said, some studies have linked fluoridation of water to having a detrimental effect on developing cells of the immune system and bone cells. On the other hand, there are many studies that show scientists proved no cell destruction and came up with the greatness of fluoridation of water.

With that said, there was and still is a lot of money being put into the fluoridation of water with a lot of lobbyists doing what they do best. It definitely fights tooth decay, but so does brushing and flossing. So I have to ask, why are you forcing this chemical on me? We still do not know what is causing so many people to have Cancer; we can only assume the possibilities and try to prevent Cancer by eliminating the possibilities or the high probabilities.

Remember that it has been said by many people that are against the fluoridation of water that fluoride has been linked to damaging the cells of the immune system. You do not have to believe in conspiracy theories, just simply do the math and make the decision as to whether or not you are going to allow your family to digest this chemical all day, every day. Most of your filters in the refrigerator do not remove the fluoride and many other unwanted chemicals.

You need to drink a lot of water and it needs to be good chemical free water. I am giving you my opinion and what I strongly believe will keep you and your family safe. We don't know what's causing all the Cancer. I believe (without a shadow of a doubt) that the more chemicals you allow in your system, the more they contribute not only to Cancer but a weaker immune system. This opens the door to a magnitude of other diseases and medical conditions.

Chapter 9
Processed Food and
Highly Processed Food

There is a big difference between processed food and highly processed food. Processed food can be classified as basic, canning, freezing, baking or drying. So of course you can eat processed food, but be aware that highly processed food is not healthy for you.

Highly processed means it can only be made in a lab or by a chemical process like with high fructose corn syrup (HFCS), or hydrogenated oil, soy protein isolate or Aspartame. These are the ingredients you should avoid as these chemicals are used to produce highly processed foods.

At the beginning of my journey of healthy living, I was frustrated because everything seemed to be processed. It got to the point that everything I was doing was wrong. Well, I do not want you to get frustrated, so I am going to tell you that it is ok to eat processed food. This chapter is going to key in on processed foods and tell you the ones to eat and the ones to stay away from because there is a huge difference between processed and highly processed foods.

This is not a Diet, Rather it is a Sensible Way to Eat Healthy

I want to try and key in on eating healthy without a lot of diet type rules. If I had to pick a diet out there—it would be a clean high protein diet. Paleo is a good choice if you are looking for a diet. Sorry Paleo, but Grain is good when eaten properly. I do however understand that too much grain is terrible for you and that you should only eat whole grain. Most of the bread out there is not whole grain; so, I agree with them, it is unhealthy. Gluten causes a lot of people various different medical problems and others it does not affect at all. Use caution and pay attention to your body.

Can I Eat Processed Food and be Healthy?

The answer to that question is yes you can. You can not only be healthy, but you can be extremely healthy. This book is based on sensible eating and trying to restrict sensibility just does not make sense. We are going to start with grain and the big differences.

Very Important when Eating Bread

Most bread is processed and unhealthy. With that said, we simply buy whole grain organic bread. The grain is intact. When the grain is left intact it contains the bran and the germ which is where your vitamins are. Without the grain intact, there are literally no vitamins to speak of. When buying grain, look for keywords like WHOLE GRAIN or WHEAT GERM. Look for organic bread with those keywords. Usually, whole grains are good. Making sure it is organic assures you that unhealthy chemicals are not used while processing.[16] This is huge!

The same thing goes for cereal. Organic cereal is processed but not chemically processed. While we are talking cereal I will mention the same goes for almond milk. Organic almond milk is not processed with the food additive carrageenan (substance thickener) which can cause some people food allergies. It is my opinion that if you buy Organic when eating processed foods you are not crossing the fine line to highly processed food. This can be a good rule of thumb when shopping.

When shopping for oatmeal look for rolled oats and steel cut oats. They are filled with fiber, metabolism boosting folate, and muscle friendly phosphorus

On the Other Hand

Instant oatmeal or microwavable oatmeal are equivalent to a captain crunch type cereal. These are some examples of the difference between processed and highly processed foods.

If you are sensitive to grain, consult your doctor. Everyone else can go ahead and enjoy your grain but remember that too much is not good. Always make sure your grain is a "carrier of goodness" and you fill that grain with great nutrients like seeds, bananas and almonds to name a few. That is the

---

[16] Organic Bread Versus "Natural" And Conventional Bread, PlanetSave, Sept 20, 2012, https://planetsave.com/2012/09/20/organic-bread-versus-natural-and-conventional-bread/

key in my opinion. Pack your grains with all the goodness I list in Chapter 12, Get Your Nutrients on the Go.

Recap

Make sure when you buy grain its whole grain, whole wheat, brown rice or rolled oats. If not, the product is simply unhealthy and possibly causing you harm.

Highly Processed Food: Worth Mentioning Again

Highly processed means it can only be made in a lab or through a chemical process like with high fructose corn syrup (HFCS), or hydrogenated oil, soy protein isolate or aspartame. When you see these ingredients, it is surely highly processed. Highly processed food is suggested to be a contributor to our world's major medical problems that everyday people have.[17] It is my personal opinion these foods should not even be allowed to be made. They are terrible for you.

Food for Thought

According to IARC (International Agency for Research on Cancer) one hot dog a day is enough to increase your risk of Colorectal Cancer by 18%![18] Their main objective is to evaluate

---

[17] The Many Health Risks of Processed Foods, Laborers Health & Safety Fund of North America, May, 2019, https://www.lhsfna.org/index.cfm/lifelines/may-2019/the-many-health-risks-of-processed-foods/#:~:text=Heavily%20pro-cessed%20foods%20often%20include,Lacking%20in%20nutritional%20value

[18] Hot Dogs are now considered carcinogens by the IARC, Washingtonpost.com, Oct 26, 2015, https://www.washingtonpost.com/news/to-your-

the carcinogenicity of an agent to humans. In this case, the agent was hot dogs and of course all the chemicals it takes to process and fill the hotdog.

Read the Ingredients: The 12 Worst Chemicals

When shopping it is very important to read the labels and particularly the ingredients. Below are the 12 worst chemicals that I want you to look for and avoid. They are the chemicals in the highly processed foods that we need to avoid. I encourage you to have this list as they are in so many of our foods and most likely throughout your pantry. Keeping in mind they cause a host of medical problems like diabetes, obesity and Cancer.

1. MSG- monosodium glutamate - Linked to harmful neurological effects and impaired growth.
2. Artificial food coloring, Food Dye – Linked to Thyroid tumors, ADHD - Potential Cancer causing effects.
3. Sodium Nitrate – Deli Meats - Linked to several types of Cancer.
4. Guar Gum found in ice cream and soups – Linked to bloating, cramps, intestinal blockage and gas.
5. HFCS (High Fructose Corn Syrup) found in soda, candy, etc. - Associated with weight gain, morbid obesity, diabetes, and inflammation of cells! It also causes acne and speeds up the aging process.
6. Artificial Sweeteners (aspartame, sucralose, saccharin and acesulfame potassium) – Causes headaches and a lot more.

health/wp/2015/10/26/hot-dogs-are-now-considered-carcinogens-here-are-roughly-480-other-things-the-who-says-might-cause-cancer/

7. Carrageenan, creamers – Associated with Ulcers, Growths, High Blood Sugar, Colitis.
8. Sodium Benzoate (fruit juices) – Cancer development, ADHD, increased hyperactivity.
9. Trans Fat found in margarine, microwave popcorn – inflammation which is a major risk factor of heart disease and possible connection to Diabetes.
10. Xanthan Gum, found in dressings and soups causes digestive problems.
11. Artificial Flavoring - animal studies showed decreased red blood cell production.
12. Yeast Extract (High sodium) - soy sauce, salty snacks – headaches, numbness and swelling.

All of these have been linked to some of our everyday medical conditions, including minor problems like headaches up to and including heart conditions and Cancer.

Reality in a Busy World

There are a lot of the foods I mentioned and suggested to eat that are processed. But if you Buy Organic and watch your ingredients, you will notice they do not fall into the highly processed area. This is what you want to stay away from. In Chapter 12, Get Your Nutrients on the Go, you are again using some processed grains to carry all your real food super foods. This is the key to processed food.

The foods listed below all fall into being Highly Processed and many of them are linked to Cancer. Again, we do not know for sure what is causing all the Cancer, but several of the below foods are linked to Cancer and a multitude of medical conditions.

Please try to avoid the Following:

- Potato Chips
- Cakes and Pastries
- Bacon, Sausage, Hot dogs and Deli Meats
- Soda
- Milk

Remember this is a lifelong journey. Don't get discouraged. The first step is starting to think about people's everyday ailments and evaluate if they can be linked to their diet. We can't avoid all of the processed foods all of the time but we can avoid the highly processed foods most of the time. Be on guard and pay attention to the physical ailments that these chemicals can cause. Try finding healthier alternatives instead. I promise making these changes will promote a happier, healthier life for you and your family.

Food for Thought:

Too much sugar intake and high fructose corn syrup can cause dry scalp, dandruff, hair thinning and hair loss.[19]

[19] You're Losing Hair Because of Your Diet, Not Your Genes, Joey Wakeman, Jul 8, 2019, https://medium.com/@joeywakeman/youre-losing-hair-because-of-your-diet-not-your-genes-6f40ee7191d5

Chapter 10
Organic and Non Organic

The primary reason to buy organic is to keep you and your loved ones healthy by avoiding a multitude of chemicals that may cause you and your family medical conditions:

- Genetically modified organisms (GMO)
- Hormones
- Antibiotics

Protecting Mother Earth is another important reason to buy organic. Preserve our ecosystem by keeping farmland clean with non-toxic soil.

Preserving Our Delicate Water Ways

Traditional farming uses so many insecticides, and fertilizers that are full of toxic chemicals. These chemicals seep directly into our streams, rivers and oceans poisoning our fish and animals. Organic farmers are not permitted to use these chemicals. By purchasing organic you are supporting many local farmers and protecting Mother Earth.

In this chapter I would like to bring to your attention what to buy Organic and what not to buy Organic. Not all foods need to be Organic so you can save some money if you so choose.

Organic means it must be grown without pesticides, synthetic fertilizers or sewage sludge, GMOS (Genetically Modified Organism) or Ionizing radiation. The same goes for animals that produce meat, poultry, eggs and dairy products; they must be free from antibiotics and hormones. This is great news for those who try and eat healthy.

What is Certified Organic?

Certified Organic is a registered trademark with routine and frequent random audits.

Got Poisoned Veggies?

This is a particularly important chapter as so many of us do not realize that our basic foods are literally poisoned. I mean let's not walk backwards. So many of us think we are eating healthy but unknowingly we are digesting harmful chemicals. For so long I thought I was eating healthy, but I was not. So many of our farmers use a lot of heavy pesticides, herbicides and insecticides that a basic rinse is not going to remove the poison. In fact it might be impossible to remove all the chemicals from your food.

Pesticides Cause Cancer

Imagine getting a headache or becoming nauseous after eating a fresh salad with bell pepper. The fact is, we do not know for sure what caused the headaches or nausea. We have learned (through testing), that some of our vegetables are known to have these chemicals on them. This is not something that is monitored for consumers who are ready to buy their peppers. We have always quickly washed our vegetables, with many of us thinking we just need to clean them and wash the dirt off and not thinking about removing poison. Now that we are learning more, we have realized it is not the dirt we are worried about, rather it is the poison. Many of the products absolutely need to be Organic. Big money farms are not going to lose crops to insects or weeds. They will kill them by poisoning them. The result is your produce is tainted with poison. It has hazardous chemicals that can cause Cancer and many other ailments and diseases.[20]

What is Causing All this Cancer?

What I am telling you it is very important, and you need to tell your loved ones about it. We do not know what is causing so many people to have Cancer. We do know that pesticides and herbicides are strongly linked to Cancer and considered carcinogens. So, let's not ingest them. Remember, it's not the dirt we are worried about, your immune system will fight off these simple microbes, it's the poison that works on destroying your immune system. This is why we buy organic and or soak our fruits and veggies with baking soda.

[20] Cancer health effects of pesticides, Systematic Review, Oct 2007, U.S. National Library of Medicine National Institutes of Health, https://www.ncbi.nlm.nih.gov/pmc/articles/PMC2231435/

The Dirty Dozen

All of the products below may contain heavy pesticides and buying organic is recommended. A quick wash is not sufficient. You must soak them, using a teaspoon of baking soda if not buying organic. I encourage you to have this list on your refrigerator as these fruits and vegetables are known to have high pesticide residue.

1. Apples – Heavy Pesticides. Buy Organic they are not that expensive
2. Bell Peppers – Heavy Pesticides
3. Spinach - Heavy Pesticides. Buy Organic. Note: romaine lettuce has far less pesticides than spinach
4. Kale
5. All berries including blueberries
6. Peaches
7. Cherries
8. Pears
9. Tomatoes
10. Potatoes– Sweet Potatoes have far less pesticides
11. Celery
12. Grapes

Note: This list changes as there are others so I encourage you to start becoming familiar with them and try to purchase organic. If you unable to locate organic remember to soak with a teaspoon of baking soda, then wash and rinse.

There are surely other vegetables and fruits covered with pesticides, so be smart and protect your family, and continue to do your own research. Join my Clean Living Club on YouTube and watch my videos. Here I will promote some quality companies producing farmed raised animals and vegetables.

The Clean 15

Now on a Positive Note:

In theory, we are taught thick skinned, peelable fruit and veggies are on the safe side. With that said you do not have to buy these products organic unless of course you prefer the taste. Or maybe you want to do your part protecting Mother Earth. Let's start with ABCs (1-5 below). The first 7 are in my diet 3 to 4 times a week. All are high in nutrients and clean.

1. Avocado
2. Asparagus
3. Broccoli
4. Cabbage
5. Cauliflower
6. Onions
7. Mushrooms
8. Melons
9. Papaya
10. Sweet Potatoes
11. Kiwi
12. Mangos
13. Eggplants
14. Watermelons
15. Organic frozen blueberries

When I started the journey, I took a long look at all the vegetables out there and then of course looked at the Clean 15 and The Dirty Dozen I decided it was in our best interest to eat the vegetables with the least amount of pesticides and herbicides and that were packed with nutrition. Asparagus, broccoli, cauliflower and cabbage cook great together on low heat cast iron with coconut or olive oil. All 4 are packed with nutrients and have a crunchy texture so leftovers are great. Make sure you don't overcook and cook enough for 3 days. They reheat nicely and are just as good or better on day 2!

What about Meat?

Personally, I am a lot more critical of meat because of hormones and antibiotics being added which is causing our country a host of medical problems like obesity.

As I stated earlier, Organic food labeling is wonderful news for the consumer. Organic assures us that animals that produce meat, poultry, eggs and dairy products must be free from antibiotics and hormones. This is great news for those of us who try and eat healthy. Look for a stamped complete circle with a brown circumference and a half white and green colored inner. It will say USDA in green lettering and white background and ORGANIC in white lettering and green background. If it does not have this stamp it is not organic.[21]

Being Critical of Meat

Beware of Feeding of The Masses. No one said this journey was going to be easy. Finding clean meat is one of the

---

[21] Organic 101: What the USDA Organic Label Means, U.S. Department of Agriculture, Mar 13, 2019, https://www.usda.gov/media/blog/2012/03/22/organic-101-what-usda-organic-label-means

biggest challenges. I just want to bring a few things to your attention. A Chicken Farm is one of the nastiest things you will see. I encourage you to do your own study on these foods and don't believe because it's Green this or Green that it is healthy. It may be the lesser of two evils. Cage free only means there are literally thousands upon thousands of chickens in a barn able to fight each other, which causes disease, infections, and injury. They do not have enough room, and millions of chickens die each year in this type of environment. I also encourage you to watch the movie *Food Inc.* It is an older video, but little in the industry has changed. With that said, I am going to write a book on our meat processing system and the feeding of the masses.

I encourage all of you to step outside the box when it comes to your meat.

I Need Protein - But Bleached Meat?

Even if you can get past the filthiness of the slaughter-houses you cannot get past all the chemicals used in the process, including a chlorinated bath for chickens. It is Government mandated. Yes, that is correct. Your Green and Blue smart chickens are soaked in chlorine because they are covered with bowels their entire life. It is in my opinion buyer beware. We do not know what is causing all the Cancer in the world. We do know that chlorine and bleach are linked to Cancer. Do we know if they were properly rinsed? Or maybe they skipped that step because the well paid farm hand was in a rush. The bottom line is that there is too much room for error for me.

I Love Meat – But Vegetarian?

I totally understand one of the main concepts of our vegetarian friends. The meat processing is tainted. So, my suggestion to you is to always wash your meat. Many say not to because it might cause salmonella or other illnesses. Do not listen to them. Just be careful and mindful as you wash the dirty bird, you want to make sure most of the bleach is off. I personally buy our chickens from a local farmer who raises and processes them properly. We also buy beef and pork from local farmers who take pride in the production process. These farmers are out there and in my opinion you should take the time to find quality meat. I know these animals are not only fed properly but the entire process is to bring quality food to the market. This is a good example of stepping outside the box. I have removed myself from feeding of the masses as far as meat goes. I encourage you to do the same.

Store Bought Grass Fed Beef

I do buy organic ground beef and steaks on a regular basis from our supermarkets. Making sure they have the green and white seal. Don't be discouraged when people say things like. "All cows are grass fed", or some might say "Well it's still a beef slaughterhouse".

They are correct on both accounts but are forgetting about the main reason why regular beef makes people sick and causes obesity which is linked to Cancer and weakens the immune system. These meats are not pumped with antibiotics and hormones. That is the main reason to buy the grass fed but more importantly labeled organic. From the research I have done the slaughter-house may be the same for the organically fed cow but it is a completely different animal.

I encourage you to go to local farmers to buy most of your meat if possible. If not, try and buy organic and remember to wash your meat no matter what you read, especially the chlorinated birds

---

Bon Appétit

Join my Clean Living Club and watch my videos. Here I will promote some quality companies producing great products. Also some great places in Florida where to buy quality raised animals for good clean chicken, beef and pork.

Clean Living Club With Nicky P:
https://www.youtube.com/channel/UCd4mH8mA4Y8rtXK1_RHC09Q

Chapter 11
Big Switches

In this chapter I want to bring to focus on some changes we should make as we continue to learn how to build our immune system and not weaken it. If you can make the majority of these changes I am certain that you are learning how to be strong from the inside, which is first and foremost. Your outward physical condition will follow in a natural way and then your desire to stay fit will be brought forward. You will begin to follow your body's lead whether it be yoga, weight lifting or just walking.

By getting your balanced diet in order all of your body's systems will work in harmony producing a well-oiled machine. Some of you are already physically fit and will feel even better and some will dive right into working out after taking my suggestions. For those of you who are not physically fit right now I just want to make sure you do not get discouraged, because your desire will change naturally and I promise you will look and feel healthier if you can implement most of my suggestions.

Let's get on with these Big Switches and see how many you can implement in your life. Making these changes is an easy way to start living a cleaner and healthier Life. So, without further ado here are the Big Switches I recommend.

- Bottled water OUT
- Filtered water IN

- Milk Chocolate OUT
- 70% Dark Chocolate IN (Actually healthy and full of antioxidants)
- High heat cooking OUT
- Low heat cooking IN (Reduces toxins)
- Non stick cookware and aluminum OUT.
- Cast Iron Stainless Steel IN (Actually increases daily iron intake)
- Added Sugar OUT
- Sugar OUT
- Stevia or Raw Honey IN
- Mayo and Catsup OUT
- Mustard IN
- Household cleaners OUT
- Water and Vinegar IN
- Deli and Domestic meat OUT
- Organic Meat IN (Ethically raised animals preferred)
- Farm raised fish and shrimp OUT
- Local market Shrimp and fish IN (Avoid buffets and all you can eat. Mostly all farm raised and toxic)
- Peanut Butter OUT
- Almond Butter IN (Reduce your cholesterol)
- Dairy Milk OUT
- Organic Almond or Coconut milk IN
- All margarine OUT
- Real Butter IN (Good fat)
- White Potatoes OUT (White potatoes are not bad for you unless you pack it with junk)
- Sweet potatoes IN (Sweet potatoes have more nutrients, less pesticides)
- Tomato Paste OUT
- Organic tomato sauce IN
- Pasta OUT

- Whole grain pasta IN (Its processed but a healthier choice)
- Most all bread OUT
- Organic Whole Grain IN
- Plastics OUT
- Glass and stainless IN
- Antiperspirant OUT
- Natural organic deodorant or essential oils IN
- Apples OUT
- Organic Apples IN
- Bell peppers OUT
- Organic Bell Peppers IN (There are others but make sure peppers and apples you switch because of high pesticide usage)
- Salad dressing OUT
- Vinegar IN
- Instant oatmeal OUT
- Steel Oats Oatmeal IN
- Microwave use OUT
- Oven / Stove IN
- Lighter fluid OUT
- High flames black charcoal cooking OUT
- Low heat Gray coals IN
- Natural Flavors OUT
- Artificial Colors or Flavors OUT

What's in Your Shopping Cart?

You will learn how many products that are on the shelves of a grocery store are downright not good for you. If we were able to actually inspect people's shopping carts to see what they were buying we would come up with a rather quick con-clusion that our country has a problem. No wonder people have Diabetes, Obesity and eventually get Cancer.

The above Big Switches are strong recommendations I feel you should try to implement in you and your families households. Keeping your family healthy is the key.

Chapter 12
Get Your Nutrients
on the Go

This Chapter is dedicated to all the busy people in the world that think they do not have time to eat healthy. It may come across like I am telling you how to eat, but I am merely suggesting easy popular foods that you can prepare in minutes as they provide you the essential nutrients you need. Of course they are suggestions and I encourage you to change it up to fit your likes. Just remember, the following foods I am listing are essential, and they will make you feel great. Keeping your body happy is something you will learn. Once you start to build this healthy journey and living a healthier life your body will subtly desire the need for healthier food, rather than only satisfying your taste buds.

Organic Reminder

Before I mention the simple on the go meals, I want to re-iterate about going organic. Going organic will help prevent Cancer and support your immune system. It's a simple step in the right direction.

Pesticide Reminder

Pesticides and Insecticides cause Cancer. I want to remind you of the importance of not only eating your fruits and vegetables but soaking and washing them. Soaking your berries with a little baking soda breaks down the pesticides and removes the poisonous residue from your food. Going organic prevents you and your family from ingesting pesticides.

Are You In A Rush?
Get Your Nutrients On The Go!

Here is a great game plan for you that will fortify you with various vitamins and nutrients and is designed for you to eat on the run and/or eat quickly without a lot of preparation. Please print out or copy this list so you will always have these nutrients on hand. It is a solid core of easy access nutrients that hopefully will be on your countertop not tucked away in the cabinet. If you are just starting this journey or reading to pick up some advice let these be on your grocery list. Of course you may not like some of these and you may even change up your veggies to fit your desires. Having these nutrients always on hand will assist you as you build your immune system and become a healthier human being. Whole grains should be a carrier of your nutrients, not the main ingredient. Always remember to use your grains as your carrier of goodness.

Solid Core of Nutrients

- Seed mix, Chia, Flax and Hemp
- Oatmeal (Steel cut- Rolled Oat)
- Whole Almonds Natural and plain, Unsalted
- Crushed Almonds (Get a blender and every couple of weeks fill up your glass jar)
- Organic Cereal
- Organic Bread
- Organic Pizza

- Cauliflower Pizza
- Grass Fed Beef- Buy a lot and freeze
- Organic Almond Milk
- Organic Live Culture Yogurt
- Apple Cider Vinegar (With the mother)
- Kombucha
- Cilantro
- Avocados buy a lot. When they get older, make a smoothie with them. Never run out and never waste. They are high in nutrients
- Almond butter. Almond Butter is much healthier, but if you can't afford it, then go with all natural peanut butter instead
- Organic plant based Protein Powder
- Organic Eggs - Hard boiled eggs on the go!!!
- Organic spinach or spring garden or Romaine
- Organic apples
- Bananas - Buy Bunches. Buy green and yellow. You should eat 2 or 3 a day. When they are getting old--it is Smoothie Time!!
- Blueberries
- Mushrooms
- Onions
- Garlic
- Berries Soak Wash Rinse. Organic is pricey but NO Pesticides. Frozen Organic Blueberries are great for smoothies and oatmeal
- Organic Beet Powder
- Organic Green Powder
- Organic Bell Peppers. (All Colors. Red peppers have the highest vitamin C)
- Sweet Potatoes
- Asparagus (Your ABC's)
- Broccoli

- Cauliflower
- Cucumber
- Celery
- Ginger Powder- Ginger and Turmeric seem hard to get in my diet on a regular basis. So I buy the powder and have a cool drink or a warm tea by mixing them together
- Turmeric Powder -these two have a multitude of health benefits
- Red or White or Rice Vinegar

Now you have a core of nutritious ingredients that will literally change you. You will feel amazing and full of energy. Because we live in a busy world and many of us spend a lot of time on the go I am going to lay out a plan for you to consume these ingredients. This plan worked for me, while running a business and working a full time EMS job. I carried the load and managed to eat very healthy. It was a very stressful few years and I lived on four or five hours of sleep (which I do not recommend). But even so, I did not come close to getting sick, even while being around sick people. Why?

Because eating healthy works, and it allows your body to fight off sickness, by building your immune system and of course keeps Cancer at bay!

Breakfast in the Books in Minutes!

Ok, get your steel cut oatmeal and put 1 to 2 cups in your large double wall stainless steel cup. Add your Almond milk, avocado, blueberries, seeds, bananas and crushed almonds. Then pour boiling water in the cup and carefully stir. Put the lid on it and you have up to 3 hours to eat a nice hot breakfast (do not eat for approx. 20 minutes as the oats are still cooking).

Of course you can mix it up and add organic plant based protein powder, peanut butter powder, and/or different berries or fruits. Obviously you do not have to add all of those ingredients but put in what you can keeping in mind you should have most of these products in your diet. I will mention you cannot get enough bananas. They are so good for you and cheap. I recommend 2 or 3 a day.

You Don't Want A Hot Meal?

This is actually my favorite and not just for breakfast.

Organic cereal and crushed almonds and Organic almond milk. Add as many as the above nutrients for a cool refreshing meal. They are all important but if you just want to add a few go with banana, blueberries and crushed almonds and seeds.

Snack Time

Organic apples are a perfect snack. You can always have a few handfuls of almonds, or maybe a banana or a hardboiled egg.

Lunch Time on the Go

If you are on the go, maybe go with a sandwich with organic bread of course. I like to make organic beef patties and leave a few in the refrigerator for quick meals. Sweet potato wedges are great to have on hand. They last a few days contained in the refrigerator.

My Favorite: another delicious option is an almond butter sandwich on organic bread. I like adding a banana, crushed almonds and blueberries and more seeds please!!

You are again stacked with nutrients! Change it up and some days go with sliced egg and avocado. They are all so nutritious. This meal is so easy to take with you on the go, much like your oatmeal or cereal for that matter.

Snack Time Again

It is ok to eat a lot when you are eating good things. Your metabolism will improve as you continue to eat healthy and you most likely will be very active because you have good clean energy to burn.

Smoothie Time!

This could be a meal on the go. Suit yourself of course. This is where your organic live culture yogurt comes in, along with a little almond milk. Now throw in a handful of crushed almonds, and avocado and another banana, (LOL) and some organic protein powder if you like. Don't forget to add more seeds. It is so easy to make and very good for you. Use your imagination and fulfill your desires with your likes!

Dinner Time on the Go

I enjoy Pizza maybe a couple times a week. Remember that grain is a carrier of goodness. Organic and cauliflower pizzas are delicious, but they need additional ingredients. Top your frozen pizza with onion and minced garlic. Maybe add some mushrooms and for sure add some pre-cooked grass fed ground beef (that you prepped for the week). Add more seeds!

Dinner will be complete with a small salad. If you get burnt out on salads (which many people do), I suggest you mix it up. You do not always have to have greens. They are great for you, but I know people tend to not want greens every day. I suggest you go with bell peppers and cucumbers one day and celery and onions the next. You get the idea, mix it up. Keep in mind that greens are essential and they are filled with goodness that keeps you in balance.

Another Food for Thought

Did you know thin cut broccoli stalks on your pizza are not only very nutritious but delicious and crunchy? Most people throw them away and they hold the majority of the nutrients.

OH NO! In a JAM?

If and when you find yourself in a situation and you are hungry and the only option is a gas station or a friend's house or any other compromising situation you may slip up and eat some unhealthy foods. Do not get discouraged, you will get back on track. Stay sensible. Some gas stations have organics.

Some of them have almonds, eggs, salads and maybe a quality protein bar. We all slip up, and it's not a big deal. Most of you will still eat cake but hopefully only at birthday parties. If you cheat with chips, I recommend organic corn chips. Salsa is good for you! Don't get discouraged if you go off track.

Getting all of your nutrients and not putting in unwanted harmful chemicals is essential for your body and mind to function properly. Your body is made up of several systems but delivering superfoods to your digestive tract is of the utmost of importance as it feeds the remaining systems so they function properly. If you properly maintain your digestive tract you will run better than a well-oiled machine. This complete circle of mental and physical health fights off viruses and prevents Cancer. That is what we are doing here, and you and your family will reap the rewards. Your brain and your body work as a team. They communicate with each other and create emotions. Your complete well-being depends on how well you feed it and not compromise it.

Now you are eating healthy on the go!!!

Chapter 13
Protein Power

In my opinion, protein is the most essential nutrient you need to add to your diet to start your healthy journey. I am not going to go in depth on all the wonderful nutrients, but protein is a must have. I encourage you to start eating good quality protein, and now I will tell you why.

What is Protein?

Protein is a substance that has amino acids, compounds and carbon, hydrogen, oxygen and nitrogen. Your body uses proteins to build and repair tissues. It also uses protein to produce enzymes, hormones and other natural body chemicals. I can tell you this through first-hand knowledge. When I started this wonderful journey, I had a few bad habits--including soda and coffee (I still drink coffee, but black and organic.) I knew I needed to stop this cycle, but I liked the way the coffee and soda gave me a lift. I started exercising and (by talking to others) learned protein is a good source to aid muscle development. I started out with protein drinks like Muscle milk, protein bars, etc. I then started to eat a lot of good protein including nuts, eggs, and of course meat. Thus I made the Big Switch to include a lot of protein in my diet easier. Protein not only fills the void of soda and coffee, but you immediately start to feel healthier.

Overweight or Skinny?

My recommendation to you is to start eating good quality protein like organic eggs, grass fed beef hamburgers and almonds. Also, if you are on the go, eating protein bars can be an option. Organic plant- based protein powder is another good option. Take it every day until you get in the swing of things as your high protein daily intake becomes natural. You can take it before or after you work out or as a meal supplement or snack. I want to reiterate - go with the plant-based organic powder. It is processed but you will get on the right track and your body will love you for it. This is much better than some of the body builder type powders. There are a lot of not so healthy ingredients in those powders, so use caution. I have done a lot of the foot work through trial and error, so you don't have to.

If you are overweight and sluggish or skinny and weak, it is my opinion that good quality protein is what you are looking for. It will help you kick the sodas and energy drink habits even if you choose not to work out. Put good quality protein in your diet right away. I suggest that you intake protein at least 3 times a day and the more the better. Start to focus on putting good quality protein in every meal. Some studies suggest that too much protein can lead to kidney stones. This very well might be due to a combination of poor fluid intake and alcohol consumption. My opinion is that you cannot get enough protein in your diet. Everyone metabolizes differently, and again I feel you have nothing to worry about but always consult your doctor.

Medical Benefits

Studies Show That:[22]

Protein lowers your blood pressure. A lot of good protein in your diet is known to decrease high blood pressure. There is a good chance you may be able to come off your blood pressure medication with this healthier high protein intake and of course some other good recommendations (under your doctor's supervision).

Protein lowers your bad cholesterol which means it is good for your heart. Studies also show protein increases your metabolism and increases fat burning.

Protein helps with weight loss. Protein makes you feel full with less food. This curbs your appetite. Protein removes the hunger hormone Ghrelin which prevents cravings, and finally, protein helps with Diabetes Type 2. And for our underweight thin people who need more meat on their bones, protein will not only create muscle mass for you but help you gain weight.

In a Nutshell, Protein:

- Decreases blood pressure
- Decreases cholesterol
- Aids in controlling obesity
- Aids in controlling or eliminating diabetes

---

[22] 10 Science-Backed Reasons to Eat More Protein, Healthline, Kris Gunnars, Mar 8, 2019, https://www.healthline.com/nutrition/10-reasons-to-eat-more-protein

These are a few of our world's major medical problems. I feel that a high protein diet will assist you on your healthy living journey.

Got Sex?

Essentially, protein is a vital source for a healthy lifestyle, not to mention it just flat out makes you feel strong and creates a long-lasting energy. And that's the best news of all. Well almost.

Protein is a key substance needed to produce testosterone.[23] Ok ladies and gentlemen, it is time to put your spouse on a high protein diet. Keep it as clean as you can, by eating organic beef and eggs, and always have good nuts and seeds nearby. Do your research and listen to your body. It will start communicating with your brain and you will know what your body likes. Enjoy your life by adding a high protein intake!

---

[23] 8 Proven Ways to Increase Testosterone Levels, Healthline, Rudy Mawer, May 20, 2016, https://www.healthline.com/nutrition/8-ways-to-boost-testosterone#_noHeaderPrefixedContent

Chapter 14
Food Additives and Preservatives to Avoid

Added Sugar

Sugar side effects are also obesity, diabetes and heart disease. Just avoid added sugar.[24]

Sugar and High Fructose Corn Syrup

HFCS is in so many of Americas most purchased products. HFCS is terrible for you and your family and could possibly lead to obesity and diabetes. And just because you are thin and metabolize quickly, it does not mean you will not be affected by this chemical process. It is not good for your heart and causes vascular disease. There are a lot of other side effects from sugar and HFCS that are not talked about. Did you or your children seek medical attention with a skin specialist for having an acne problem? Maybe you were prescribed some expensive medication that has a list of side effects. If this is true and your families diet was not brought up in conversation you should reconsider your choices in physicians. Parents, you need to look at the ingredients your family is ingesting. HFCS also is linked to cell damage. In many conditions cell

---

[24] The sweet danger of sugar, Harvard Health Publishing, Nov 5, 2019, https://www.health.harvard.edu/heart-health/the-sweet-danger-of-sugar#:~:text=%22The%20effects%20of%20added%20sugar,Hu

damage is worse than cell death. A damaged cell is still alive and can become Cancerous.

Here is a list of products that contain HFCS with my alternative suggestions:

- Soda - Drink clean water with lemon slice, apple cider vinegar or organic green teas
- Candy- Go 70% Dark Chocolate
- Yogurts - Buy organic with live cultures
- Salad dressing – Don't put something bad on something good, use vinegar
- Frozen foods and TV dinners and pizza. Go organic frozen, yes it's processed but healthier
- Breads - Go organic and whole grain
- Canned Fruit – Buy real fruit
- Juice - Only drink a little and make sure it does not contain added sugar or HFCS
- Granola Bars - Look for whole grain
- Cereal - Buy Organic, It is processed but without harmful ingredients
- Snack Foods - Almonds
- Condiments - Learn to like Mustard
- Sugar and HFCS -Are slow killers. Please avoid as this is a huge step on your new journey

YOU CAN DO IT!

Trans Fats

Trans Fats are by far the worst of all the fats. They are linked to Cancer, diabetes and heart disease. Eliminating ingestion of Trans Fats is another big step in living a cleaner life.

Trans Fats are the high cholesterol culprit that leads to strokes and heart attacks. They are also linked to diabetes and obesity which is linked to Cancer.[25] The following is a strong recommendation of foods you should avoid to get on a path of healthier eating:

- Fried Food - AVOID. A lite stir fry on low heat is good
- Margarine/Shortening- USE butter. It is real food and a healthy good fat in moderation
- Crackers - AVOID - Grab some nuts
- Microwavable Popcorn– Grab some nuts. Microwavable popcorn not only contains trans-fat but other carcinogens. Avoid and remove from your family's diet
- Donuts/Cakes/Pies - AVOID Buy dark chocolate 70%

Artificial and Natural and Artificial Colors

Artificial and Natural Flavors and Artificial Colors - This is a blanket term referring to over 100 possible chemical additives. All of them are not proven harmful but many have been. It is my opinion and the opinion of many that they are harmful to you and your family. Some should not even be allowed on the market shelves. In fact several colors and flavors were finally banned in the USA although their cousins are still infiltrating our food supply. Many of the banned colors were proven to cause ADD and ADHD.[26] How long will it be before they realize many more should be banned? Where does that leave you now? I mean food dye just sounds wrong. So they

---

[25] Dietary Trans Fatty Acid Intake in Relation to Cancer Risk: A Systematic Review, https://ascopubs.org/doi/abs/10.1200/jgo.18.45900

[26] Feed Your Child's Focus: ADHD Diet, Food Dyes & Attention, Health, Food & Nutrition, https://www.additudemag.com/feed-your-childs-focus-adhd-diet-nutrition/

call it coloring, oh, that doesn't sound bad. I encourage you not to buy products that have food dye or coloring. Some of the coloring was linked to behavioral problems and who is to say they do not cause depression and anxiety and who knows what else? Not only is this a key indicator you are eating fake non-nutritious food but it is my hope you begin to realize our main food chain is slowly poisoning you and your family possibly causing Cancer and a lot of other medical conditions.

Artificial Sweeteners

Below is a short list of several chemicals that are the main ingredients in artificial sweeteners. They are in many of our favorite foods. I highly recommend avoiding these chemicals.

- Aspartame – Found in sugar free soda, ice cream and candy affects the nervous system causing headaches, dizziness, memory loss and confusion.
- Sucralose – Found in Splenda decreases good bacteria in the gut. This opens the door to many medical ailments.
- Acesulfame Potassium found in toothpaste, mouthwash, dairy products and may cause Cancer.
- Saccharin – Artificial sweetener proven to cause Cancer in animals.
- Monosodium Glutamate (MSG) - MSG is used to enhance flavor.

More on MSG

Do you have Chest Pain? Well you might if you eat enough food that is flavored up with MSG. You also might get heart palpitations. Nitrates and too much sodium can also bring on heart palpitations. This is definitely on the avoid list. Not that I see any links to Cancer, but it causes a host of medical ailments that I am sure have sent thousands and thousands of people to the emergency room. Here are a few known side effects. The FDA HAS RECIEVED MANY ANECDOTAL REPORTS OF ADVERSE REACTIONS TO FOODS CONTAINING MSG. However their researchers have found no definitive evidence between MSG and these symptoms. Don't believe them. The FDA considers adding MSG to foods "Generally recognized as safe". DON'T BELIEVE THEM.

The following list is known as the MSG Symptom Complex.

Known side effects of MSG include[27]:

- Headache
- Flushing
- Sweating
- Facial Pressure
- Numbness and tingling and burning to face neck and other areas
- Rapid Heart Rate
- Chest pain
- Nausea
- Weakness

---

[27] What is MSG? Is it bad for you? Mayo Clinic, Katherine Zeratsky, https://www.mayoclinic.org/healthy-lifestyle/nutrition-and-healthy-eating/expert-answers/monosodium-glutamate/faq-20058196

Preservatives

A preservative is defined as "A Substance used to preserve foodstuffs, wood, or other materials against decay". I don't know about you but that just does not sound good. Salt and alcohol are the oldest preservatives KNOWN and they are not the problem in our country. The preservatives below are in many of our popular highly processed food. I encourage you to have such a list on your refrigerator until you have it memorized. These lists have been around for a long time and a simple search engine will give you great information. In my opinion this is like a well-kept secret. I mean most of the public is aware these preservatives are used but I do not think they understand the ramifications that can occur after consuming these preservatives for long periods of time. It baffles me that we generally think it is okay preserve food. It is my opinion that our health experts do not discuss the harm that preservatives cause nearly enough. They are unhealthy and harmful to you and your family.[28]

Preservatives to avoid include:

- Tert-Butylhydroquinone (TBHQ) TBHQ is put in many snack crackers, oils, noodles, and frozen foods with high concentrations in frozen fish. It is known to cause vision disturbances. It is also known to cause nausea and vomiting in laboratory animals. TBHQ causes liver

---

[28] Here's how eating artificial preservatives can affect your health, Global News, Meghan Collie, Aug 22, 2019, https://globalnews.ca/news/5792891/artificial-preserv-atives-affect-health/#:~:text=Are%20artificial%20preserva-tives%20bad%20for,our%20diets%2C%E2%80%9D%20she%20said

enlargement, neurotoxic effects, convulsions, Tinnitus, and paralysis.

- POLYSORBATE - Can cause infertility, immunosuppressant and severe allergic reactions. You will find polysorbate in ice cream, sherbet, whipped toppings and other frozen desserts.
- BHT/BHA (BUTYLATED HYDROXYANISOLE) - Is known to cause kidney stones. Also, BHA is a known carcinogen that is in so many foods it is hard to avoid. Beer, chips, snacks, cereals and flavoring agents.
- SODIUM BENZOATE- Known carcinogen. Studies suggest it will increase your risk of inflammation, obesity and ADHD. You will find this preservative in carbonated drinks, fruit juices and salad dressings.
- SULFATES – They can cause allergy like reactions and wheezing. Asthma patients use extra caution. They are also in so many foods causing people medical problems I am sure. They are found in gravies, soup mixes, canned vegetables, chips and a whole lot more.

Chapter 15
Medical Conditions
Caused By a Poor Diet

The Circle Goes Round and Round

In the upcoming chapters we will learn that several medications we take that are prescribed by our doctors to help us have not so nice side effects that can actually cause you to have a new medical condition that you will possibly be taking more medications for. We need to make note and remember that Hypertension, Diabetes Type 2 and High Cholesterol are all pretty much caused by eating poorly.

Below is a list of medical conditions caused by a poor diet. This list was put together by Dr. Tiwet, an Internal Medicine physician at <u>Advocate Lutheran General Hospital </u>in Park Ridge, Illinois.

"The medical complications that result from poor eating habits and being overweight or obese, or even just carrying too much fat in your abdominal region, are not as widely known or understood," she says.

27 Medical Issues Caused by a Poor Diet

Dr. Tiwet names 27 medical issues that a poor diet and obesity are known to cause, or are highly suspected to contribute to[29]:

1. Hypertension (high blood pressure)
2. Alzheimer's Disease/Dementia
3. Coronary Heart Disease
4. Stroke
5. Gallbladder Disease
6. Osteoarthritis
7. Sleep Apnea
8. Respiratory Problems
9. Endometrial Cancer
10. Breast Cancer
11. Prostate Cancer
12. Colon Cancer
13. Dyslipidemia (an abnormal amount of lipids, or fat, in the blood)
14. Nonalcoholic Steatohepatitis (liver inflammation caused by a buildup of fat in the liver)
15. Insulin Resistance
16. Asthma
17. Hyperuricemia (an abnormally high level of uric acid in the blood)
18. Reproductive Hormone Abnormalities
19. Polycystic Ovarian Syndrome
20. Impaired Fertility

---

[29] These 27 medical problems are caused by a poor diet, health enews, https://www.ahchealthenews.com/2017/10/24/27-medical-problems-caused-poor-diet/

21. Adult Onset Diabetes (Type 2)
22. Depression
23. Anxiety
24. Low energy levels/fatigue
25. Tooth decay
26. Acne
27. Digestive health issue

Many forms of Cancer start to develop long after the medical condition you developed from eating poorly like diabetes and obesity. Other forms of Cancer develop from the long term use of certain ingredients and chemicals we put in our systems. The point I am trying to make is that eating poorly causes the above medical conditions that may only be a sign that Cancer will develop in the future.

Chapter 16
Medications Causing
Medical Conditions

Working as a Paramedic and transporting patients for a span that covered 3 decades I became very familiar with hundreds of medications. Unfortunately, I did not begin to realize the damaging effects these medications were having on people until near the end of my career when I started my healthy living journey. I then started to pay close attention to the side effects. It was my job to pay attention to the side effects of medications but I then started digging deeper. I started questioning why so many people were taking so many medications and paying attention to the complaints they were having in relationship with the medications.

I discovered they were taking medication to counteract the side effects of other medications. Then discovering the majority of the medical ailments for many of their ER visits were because of their poor diet. Follow me here. Millions of people are actually taking medications for the side effects of other medications and that the initial medication was being taken because of their poor eating habits.

Stop the Madness

As I transported patients oftentimes I was familiar with the patient as I had previously taken them to the Emergency room. Other times the transport time was long and I was able to talk at length with my patient and ask my own investigative questions that weren't necessarily relevant to an emergency situation and might not be relevant to the receiving physician. I later discovered many of our conversations were at the beginning of my healthy living journey and was a reason why I started to think about writing this book.

Unfortunately, Emergency rooms are not designed for preventive medicine. The ER doctor generally did not want to hear me tell him that the patient was taking too many medications unless the medications pertained to the patient's chief complaint. The ER doctor already knows that the patient is probably taking too many medications but technically it is not his position as it would be the patient's primary doctor's responsibility. Well, because of the patient's diet he has several doctors and often uses the ER for one also. Another medication prescribed is the probable outcome.

Big Pharma – Not a Conspiracy Theory

I am not going to elaborate too much on the topic of Doctors prescribing too many medications as it could be the title of another book. I will touch base on it because it involves you and your loved ones health. First of all, kickbacks are illegal. On the other hand it is not illegal for Big Pharma to pay doctor fees for speaking and consulting. Also Physicians fees may include meals, travel and more. I cannot recall how many times there were spreads of foods donated to the ER staff or operating room staff by Big Pharma. Are they being kind or are they trying to get their medications used on a regular basis by a group of doctors or the hospital?

The results of a study performed in 2015 on the types of distribution of payments from industry to US Physicians found that approximately 48% of US Physicians were reported to have received a total of $2.4 billion in industry related payments.[30]

I also must mention it is no known secret that big Pharma paid doctors who prescribed more opioids than doctors who only prescribed the minimum. This is a huge problem with the ongoing opioid epidemic. But let's forget about the opioid epidemic and start to realize the same problem is and has been growing with modern day medications. Big pharma wants you to take a lot of medications. It is my opinion there are millions of people taking medications they do not need to be taking. I encourage you to look at the meds you and your loved ones are taking and write down the side effects and be familiar with them. No one is going to do it for you and unfortunately our healthcare system is not designed to help people come off of meds. It is structured to have you take more meds.

Meds Clashing With Meds

There are so many medications that clash with other medications that create a multitude of complaints. Sometimes these conditions are easy to identify, for example, headaches or dizziness, while other side effects take time to develop. This makes it difficult for clinicians to pinpoint the cause and unfortunately it is not of great importance to them unless it is a seri-

---

[30] Types and distribution of payments from industry to physicians, JAMA Network, https://media.jamanetwork.com/news-item/types-distribution-payments-industry-physicians/

ous side effect that creates unstable vital signs. Just the headaches and dizziness alone might warrant neurological workup with an MRI and maybe a prescription for a few more meds.

I am certain that this is a scenario that continues in a vicious cycle that is never ending. In most cases if a patient is taking 5 medications (common) they have no idea if a new medication is going to clash with an older medication unless it's through trial and error. And not even then unless it has near catastrophic effects with a multitude of hospitalizations will it be brought to light. Unfortunately these findings take time.

Be Mindful of Your Meds

The following are a few of our common medical conditions and the side effects of the medications:

Common Side Effects from High Blood Pressure medications include[31]:

- Chest Pain
- Palpitations
- Headache
- Dizziness
- Diarrhea
- Depression
- Dry Mouth
- Frequent urination

---

[31] Side effects of high blood pressure medications, WebMD, Mar 21, 2019, https://www.webmd.com/hypertension-high-blood-pressure/guide/side-effects-high-blood-pressure-medications#1

- Weakness in the legs
- Cramps to legs
- Skin Irritation
- Swelling around eyes

How many people are taking another medication to treat the above side effects?

Common Side Effects from Diabetes Type 2 Medications:[32]

A commonly used diabetic type 2 medication is Metformin and these are some side effects:

- Abdominal pain
- Headache
- Dizziness
- Nausea
- Vomiting
- Diarrhea
- Constipation
- Decreased Appetite
- Hypotension (Your BP may drop!)

Note: You may have Diabetes Type 2 only because of your unhealthy diet. This can be corrected.

Common Side Effects from Cholesterol Medications:[33]

You have high cholesterol because of your unhealthy diet.

---

[32] Side effects and interactions of Diabetes Drugs, WebMD, https://www.webmd.com/diabetes/diabetes-drugs-side-effects-interactions

[33] Side effects of cholesterol drugs, WebMD, https://www.webmd.com/cholesterol-management/common-side-effects-cholesterol-meds

- Diarrhea
- Constipation
- Nausea
- Vomiting
- Stomach cramps
- Muscle pain
- Headache
- Rash
- Problem sleeping

Are we taking more meds for these conditions?

Common Side effects from Antidepressants:[34]

Please note there are many more serious side effects with Antidepressants which I address in Chapter 18, Mental Health Issues.

- Weight gain because of increased appetite
- Insomnia
- Loss of Sexual Desire
- Erectile Dysfunction

Are we taking any medications for these side effects?

I hope this chapter brought to light some of the problems that exist with medications in general.

---

[34] Coping with side effects of depression treatment, WebMD, https://www.webmd.com/depression/features/coping-with-side-effects-of-depression-treatment

My suggestion to help you and your family is to avoid taking multiple medications and always consult your doctor before stopping a medication. Talk to your doctor and tell them you are going to start eating healthy and stop putting chemicals into your body. Consult with him on a game plan to come off your medications.

Note: Hypertension, Diabetes Type 2 and High Cholesterol can all be taken care of by healthy living and a healthy diet.

Chapter 17
Alcohol

How can one write a book about health without mentioning the destruction alcohol causes? I am writing this with first-hand knowledge of alcoholism and I know how it can mentally and physically cause your brain and body irreparable damage.

Alcohol Damages Cells

Putting it simply, alcohol damages cells. These damaged cells try to repair themselves which could lead to DNA changes that can be a step towards Cancer. Also, once in the body alcohol can be converted into acetaldehyde, a chemical that can damage the DNA inside cells and has been known to cause Cancer in lab animals. A healthy immune system can fight this process for many years as our body can take a lot of self-destruction, however, as time goes on serious problems may result.

Alcohol Affects Your Mindset

Mentally alcohol interferes with chemicals in the brain that are vital for good mental health. Alcohol can contribute to feelings of depression and anxiety.

Alcohol's Effects on Your Body

Consuming too much alcohol causes physical problems as well:

- HTN
- Irregular Heart rate
- Cardiomyopathy (saggy, stretched, enlarged heart), Bloating
- Obesity
- Skin flushing
- And more

Do You Make Good Decisions Drinking?

Now let's talk about decision making. Some people can drink their entire life and live a relatively healthy life and make good choices. Most cannot. I do not have any facts on this but we know that alcohol has destroyed a multitude of lives. Many people go to prison or are hospitalized, and many die way before their time. Not to mention the damage it causes loved ones, as well as the innocent victims of alcoholic behavior.

If you have a problem drinking I strongly recommend you contact your doctor and tell him you want to quit drinking. I am not going too deep here. We know alcohol can be destructive physically and mentally. It can also cause Cancer. I encourage you to take a look at your drinking and if you think you might have a problem please seek help. Help is available but you must take the first step and ask for it.

I strongly recommend you contact your doctor and tell him you want to quit drinking. It is that simple. I say to contact him in case you need help with withdrawals. Start going to AA meetings. You will meet a whole group of new friends who will give you the support you need, and you can support them as well. They have one common goal with no hidden agenda. You do not have to stop drinking to go and best of all it is FREE.

If you simply do not have the time for meetings, talk to your doctor and come up with a plan. I know people who have had success with mild antidepressants. If you go this route, use caution and don't stay on them too long (2 or 3 months) because they do have side effects that can affect your thinking.

When Alcohol Is Out, The Goodness Comes In!

Another reason I have a chapter on alcohol is that it is very difficult to try and live a healthy life while you are pouring bad chemicals into your body. Your thought process of living clean will be hindered.

Please get help if you need it.

I wish you the best!

Chapter 18
Mental Health Issues

We Have Mental Health Issues

So many of us have mental health issues. It is becoming quite alarming as millions of our working-class people are on antidepressants. This chapter focuses on mild to moderate depression, not bona fide mental illnesses such as schizophrenia, bipolar disorder, and severe depression, etc. I do not mean to downplay depression, because it is real. However, it is also a part of life that we need to overcome, and not try to live in a world of false feelings that are created by a jagged little pill. In my opinion, there are too many people taking these medications when they don't need to be. Some are making life changing decisions that they might not normally make.

Doctors prescribe these mind-altering drugs as if they were candy. You simply tell your doctor you are depressed, and it is pretty much the norm that you walk out of his or her office with a prescription that could cause you and your loved ones heartache and pain. It is not immediate in most cases; therefore, it is extremely hard to pinpoint the blame. I have witnessed loved ones have behavioral outbreaks that were not normal and their emotional angry episodes were far worse and more frequent. I have treated and transported a multitude of patients because they were suicidal or posed threats to others and the culprit might have been a new medication.

Therefore, I am talking about people who had mild to moderate depression and are now in custody of the state under a Baker's Act and arrested with a mountain of legal issues. They are now unemployed, and/or humiliated from a tiny little pill that was supposed to help them. I was fortunate to be able to talk with many of the patients during long transport times, and many of them had just begun taking this antidepressant and others abruptly stopped taking their meds. In some cases they were already taking a couple antidepressants and now they just started taking another.

What's Wrong with this Picture?

Many of our doctors are trying to fix our mental health problems with medications that have a list of side effects and other mental health side effects. In my opinion, most people do not need to be on these medications. Now, I am not a doctor, and I am not recommending you stop taking your medications. However, I do have some suggestions—and one of them is to consult with your doctor about weaning off these antidepressants.

There are many cases where people need these antidepressants because of a traumatic event like the loss of a loved one or other heart-breaking crises. In my opinion, these meds should not be permanent for someone with mild to moderate depression. What these medications are doing (in many cases) is changing the person's identity or personality. Many of the antidepressant medications work by enhancing the dopamine levels in your brain, much like alcohol without the intoxication. They make you feel good and many make you feel great. This is perfect for someone who has had a crisis and needs to function, but again, not for long periods of time.

I have both witnessed and experienced behavioral changes from the side effects of some antidepressants. These are not the normal behavior for the individual. From decision-making to sexual promiscuity that have harmed loved ones and shattered families. Many of these antidepressants have serious side effects causing mental issues with uncontrollable outbreaks of anger and continuous thoughts of suicide that often result in the worst imaginable outcome. It is my personal opinion that some of these medications are causing great harm to many.

A Game Plan for Fighting Depression with Nutrients

To boost your mental health, focus on eating plenty of fruits and vegetables along with foods rich in omega-3 fatty acids, such as salmon. Dark green leafy vegetables, in particular, are brain protective. Nuts, seeds and legumes, such as beans and lentils, are also excellent brain foods. Many studies have shown that eating a well-balanced diet reduces depression. Your brain needs the nutrients to fight depression. Equally important, your gut needs to be healthy, since your gut and brain are linked to work together through the Vagus nerve. Serotonin is a mood stabilizer, and it is believed that 95% of serotonin is produced by healthy gut bacteria. If your gut is full of bad bacteria and does not have healthy bacteria you will most likely suffer from depression.

Probiotics = Healthy Gut = No More Depression

There is another especially important reason to take a quality probiotic and to feed that probiotic with healthy prebiotics like apple cider vinegar, asparagus and onions to name a few. These 3 prebiotic foods feed your probiotic supplement, as I suggested. They then feed the good bacteria which kills the bad bacteria making your gut strong and healthy. Now you are producing a lot of Serotonin which will help you stay mentally stable so you can cope with sadness and disappointment while simultaneously channeling your good feelings with an even level of emotions.[35]

Other Nutrients Important for Your Mental Health

Nutrients such as Folate and Vitamin B6 are necessary to synthesize certain brain chemicals called neurotransmitters that regulate mood and memory. An imbalance of these neurotransmitters causes depression, anxiety and other conditions. Your ABC's: (Asparagus, Broccoli, Cauliflower) as well as Bananas and Wheat Germ is a great start

Mama Said Eat Your Greens

Well, she is right. Leafy greens, like spinach, are essential for your health and will help keep you mentally fit!!! Avocado also contains Folate which is also essential to balance your mental fitness.

---

[35] Can probiotics help with depression? Healthline, https://www.health-line.com/health/probiotics-depression#_noHeaderPrefixedContent

These Same Food Additives Cause Depression

These same food additives that were mentioned in previous chapters that cause common every day ailments also cause depression.[36] Artificial sweeteners, colors and flavors are probably the worst thing for you if you are battling depression. They are linked to ADHD and ADH and are also linked to certain types of Cancer. A list of these food additives include:

- MSG
- HFCS
- White Flour
- Tartrazine
- Hydrogenated Oils

It's a Rap

In summary, I want to make sure you consult your doctor before coming off any medication. I do encourage that you consult your Doctor and let them know you would like to possibly wean off the antidepressants. Then ask your doctor what his or her best game plan would be. Make sure you tell them you are going to keep a healthy gut and enhance your Serotonin and you will keep your Vitamin B6 and Folate in your daily diet with a quality probiotic and you will continue eating prebiotic foods. In my opinion, if he or she is a good doctor,

[36] 8 food additives sabotaging your mood, HealthCentral, https://www.healthcentral.com/slideshow/8-food-additives-sabotaging-your-mood

the practitioner will acknowledge your perseverance and encourage you, unless your mental diagnosis is not warranted
for this.

Chapter 19
Important Things to Remember

Supplemental Powders are Important

There are simply some foods that seem to be hard to incorporate into our diet, especially in a busy life on the go all the time. The good thing is that there are some great whole food powders out there to get you those vitally important nutrients. Vitamins do not hold a candle to raw powdered food. In fact, there are several reputable companies producing organic whole food powders that will allow you to be fulfilled! This is especially important for the vitamins we do not get enough of. The following are a few Organic powders that will enhance your diet, and you will feel better because you are eating healthier.

Green Leafy Powders

It is especially important to get the nutrients of Kale, Spinach and several other greens several times a week. It only takes a teaspoon in water, and you are fortified. Supplemental powders will build your immune system naturally. I find it a great way to start your day.

Organic Beet Powder

Beets are another vegetable that is essential for you to implement in your diet. Organic beet powders are available, and again, you need to have this in your diet a few times a week. This adds essential vitamins and nutrients with great health benefits to your diet. A teaspoon in water makes it easy.

Raw Ginger Organic Powder

There are so many health benefits from incorporating Ginger in your diet, since it is great for arthritis and is a natural anti-inflammatory. Ginger has been linked to improving asthma outbreaks as well. Further, Ginger is known to ease menstrual cramps and nausea. Most importantly, it curbs Cancer growth. In fact it provides an array of health benefits that might keep you off medications and out of the hospital.

Organic Turmeric Powder

Another essential nutrient that seems hard to get in your diet on a regular basis is Turmeric. The health benefits are amazing as it has potent anti-inflammatory properties. Turmeric also aids with depression and is believed to prevent Cancer, Alzheimer's, and Heart disease. Turmeric also is loaded with anti-oxidants like Ginger.

Organic Green Tea

Organic green tea is packed with health benefits as it improves brain function, it is filled with anti-oxidants that will lower your risk of Cancer. Simply buy organic powders and add them to water or mix them with green tea or however you decide to drink them. I usually combine ginger and turmeric as it creates a bold taste and offers both essential nutrients simultaneously. Once you get into the habit of drinking your tea a few times a week, you will notice the benefits right away.

So, if you live a busy life and are unable to cook I highly suggest you buy these organic powders and incorporate them into your diet. You will be amazed at how healthy you feel, and you will find that many common ailments do not show their ugly face anymore. From aches and pains, to abdominal cramping—the list of benefits goes on. More importantly they help prevent Cancer by building your Immune system.

Got Milk?

It is my opinion that milk is for baby calves. Milk is filled with various hormones that will possibly lead you to obesity. It is not the same milk many of us were raised on as it is now highly processed. Many say that milk leads to an unhealthy gut which is where most infections start. Keep your gut healthy and it will strengthen your immune system and you and your family will be less likely to get sick. Organic almond milk is a great alternative and tastes great.

Remember Your ABC'S and get Supplemental Iron

Asparagus, Broccoli and Cauliflower. These 3 superfoods cook and store well together, both before and after cooking. These superfoods do not need to be organic. I suggest cooking in a cast iron skillet with just a little coconut or olive oil and on low heat of course. Cooking in cast iron actually gives you supplemental iron intake naturally. Iron deficiency is more common in women than men.[37] Only cook for a short period of time to leave them all crunchy. These servings stay crisp and crunchy for about 4 days, and reheating is so simple.

Avoid Boiling or Frying

Boiling and frying vegetables often destroys nutrients. Be mindful of this and remember that low heat is the way to go.

The Sun is Good for You

Many people are under the impression they should not get any sun. Or perhaps, they need to soak their family with sunscreen before going out in the sun because it is documented that UV rays are harmful and can cause skin Cancer. That is true. However, I encourage you to do some research on sunscreens.

Sunscreens contain OXYBENZONE which is a known hormone disruptor and allergen.[38] This is only one of the many chemicals in sunscreen. The FDA is currently working on a new set of rules. They have finally realized these chemicals enter your bloodstream and may cause health problems. This is a definite 'buyer beware' and I encourage you to do your own investigation before coating your infant or child with sunscreen. OXYBENZONE causes male fish to turn into females.

---

[37] Why is iron deficiency anemia more common in women than in men?, Medscape Sept 30, 2020, https://www.medscape.com/answers/202333-153111/why-is-iron-deficiency-anemia-more-common-in-women-than-in-men

[38] How Safe is Your Sunscreen? American Cancer Society, Aug 9, 2018, https://www.cancer.org/latest-news/how-safe-is-your-sunscreen.html

This is a terrible hormone disruptor, and in my opinion, it is harmful to you and your family.

So what is one supposed to do? First things first. The sun is good for you. 30 minutes a day is recommended by many as you need your Vitamin D. Of course, consult your doctor, since many light-complexioned people might only want to get 10 minutes. Either way, the sun is healthy, and you should get some rays daily. If not, chances are you might become Vitamin D deficient. Using Zinc Oxide for sunscreen when you are exposed to the sun for long periods of time is recommended by many. It is a little messy, but natural and healthy. Natural sunscreens are available with a lot less harmful chemicals. Use hats, shirts and sunglasses and get an umbrella to help.

Avoid Carbon Monoxide

So many people encounter poisonous gases without realizing it. The statistics are alarming concerning accidental deaths due to gas heaters and stoves. Carbon monoxide is colorless and odorless and is a silent killer. Although the Department of Health and Human Services (DHHS) has not classified it as a carcinogen, we do know it causes headaches, dizziness, nausea and vomiting, chest pain, and confusion. This is important because you need to be cautious and aware of your surroundings whether at home with appliances or at work around machinery. Many people who are sitting in traffic breathing in carbon monoxide feel ill before they get home.

Be mindful of your surroundings everywhere you go. When in traffic, make sure you click on the "inside air" switch on your AC dashboard. Turn it too "outside air" position for open road driving only. Many people are not aware of this, and they are sucking in carbon monoxide while sitting in traffic.

There are so many harmful places and situations out there that I just wanted to bring to your attention some of the things I feel we are not fully informed of. These are little things that can cause a multitude of medical complaints and conditions leading up to, and including, Cancer.

Memory Foam – Don't Sleep with the Enemy

In my opinion, sleeping with memory foam is like sleeping with the enemy. Memory foam is an American favorite. It was created by NASA for Astronauts helmets and chairs. It soon became popular in mainstream America as it forms to your body and gives you a good night's sleep. Or so we thought. Memory foam contains toxic chemicals that are considered carcinogenic, including benzene.[39]

The International Agency for Research on Cancer classifies benzene as "carcinogenic to humans" because of strong evidence pointing to a correlation between benzene and Cancers such as acute lymphocytic leukemia and non-Hodgkin lymphoma.

Benzene is not the only toxic chemical found in memory foam. There is Naphthalene and Formaldehyde. Naphthalene causes skin and eye irritation, GI complications and even neurological symptoms. Formaldehyde is also linked to Cancer and causes headaches and skin and eye irritation. So why are

[39] Are Memory Foam Mattresses Safe? Mattress Resources, Jan 1, 2021, https://bestmattress-brand.org/are-memory-foam-mattresses-safe/

we laying our heads down on these pillows? The instructions usually direct you to "air the pillow out" if there is a foul odor. Ok, so when the toxic chemical smell is gone, does that mean there are no more chemicals to worry about? Of course there is. I encourage you to keep you and your family off these pillows and buy cotton organic pillows or even latex pillows are a safer alternative as they are not made of a cocktail of toxic chemicals. Your pillows could be causing you and your family a list of medical ailments like headaches and sinus problems and even Cancer. Please don't sleep with the enemy.

Chapter 20
Conclusion

The major objective of this book was to make you aware that if your body or mind is having some kind of ailment there is a very high probability that it is because of the chemicals you take in, whether it be from food or household and hygiene products. This is why the title of the book is PREVENT CANCER AND A LOT MORE.

Even though there appears to be a lot of overwhelming information I truly was only able to scratch the surface as I wanted to get you pointed in the right direction of living a cleaner and chemical free life.

I have provided the information you need and a course of action and game plan for you to follow as you and your family start the journey of healthier living.

There are several lists in the book that are of great importance:

- An 18 step guide to build your immune system (pages 23-24).
- A list of The Dirty Dozen fruits and vegetables to avoid unless buying organic (page 76).
- A list of the Clean 15 fruits and vegetables you should eat (page 77).
- A list of 50 Big Switches you should try to implement in your life (pages 83-85).
- The difference between processed and highly processed foods and what you should know (Chapter 9).

- A list of toxic ingredients in your household and hygiene products that you should avoid (Chapter 4).

Remember to try and eat your veggies from the clean 15, and if not make sure you buy organic. Nothing bothers me more for people being misled into thinking they are eating healthy when in essence the fruit and vegetables are coated with harmful pesticides. Many cancer patients I have spoken with thought they were eating healthy. Please don't forget the game plan for building your immune system and the importance of drinking clean chemical free water.

Please keep in mind that Big Pharma and our major food manufacturing companies are not concerned about you and your family's health. There are so many everyday ailments we are taking over the counter meds for the pharmacy loves us. That is Big Pharma and Superstores taking our hard earned money for something as simple as a poor diet.

This is why I will continue to encourage you to step outside the box and find those companies that are out there making quality products. There are more and more companies making quality products because a greater portion of society is starting to be more and more health conscious and the demand is there.

I know there are many people that will never get cancer no matter how many chemicals they take in. Many people believe that there is a gene you carry and you are susceptible or you are not. This very well may be true but regardless of this opinion even those who do not carry the gene still will suffer from many other medical conditions from A to Z. Most of these illnesses are caused by consumption of toxic chemicals and or a weak immune system. I hope in this book I was able to drive that basic concept home and you and your family can begin to realize that many of the everyday products we use are not good for us. And likewise many of the foods we were raised on are now highly processed with chemicals and filled with ingredients that are simply unhealthy (Milk and Meat).

I hope I have painted a clear picture for you that is my belief of why so many people get sick. Not only from cancer but a multitude of generalized medical conditions.

Follow me on my up and coming YouTube channel as I promise to provide you with great healthy ideas.

Join the Clean Living Club With Nicky P:
https://www.youtube.com/channel/UCd4mH8mA4Y8rtXK1_RHC09Q

In addition feel free to contact me on FaceBook and Instagram (4yorhealth).

STAY HEALTHY MY FRIENDS!

If you enjoyed this book and find it useful, please take a few moments to write a review on your favorite store, and refer it to your friends.

Appendix 1
Seasoning Your Cast Iron Cookware

Many women are Iron deficient. Using cast iron can be intimidating, and it is easy to get discouraged until you get the seasoning of the pan down. If the pan is not seasoned properly cleaning up is a mess. This is why people say no to cast iron. On the contrary, if your pans are seasoned properly, cleanup is very easy compared to other pots and pans. Scrambled eggs and cheesy things are the only things that do not clean up well. This is an easy fix by bringing water to a low boil and then wash as you normally do. Seasoning is basically giving your pan a natural slick coating.

Follow these simple steps to season your cast iron pan:

- Wash with soap and water and a scrub pad, rinse well and hand dry immediately. The only time you use soap is when seasoning.
- Coat the skillet with olive, vegetable or coconut oil. Lubricate the entire surface, even the outside.
- Bake it like a cake 30 to 45 minutes in the oven. Let cool, and you are done.
- Optional. I found this initial step helps give your pan a thicker additional coating. Take your cooled pan and add additional coconut oil and heat on a burner high for 1- 2 minutes (set your timer!).

- After each use, wash with water only and a scrub pad, hand dry and then coat with oil (buy a brush) and then reheat on high for 1-2 minutes.

Appendix 2
Per-and Polyfluoroalkyl
Substances (PFACs)

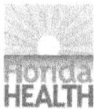

PFAS
Chemical Awareness

Florida HEALTH

Florida Department of Health · FloridaHealth.gov

Per-and polyfluorinated substances (PFAS) are a man-made family of chemicals, with PFOS (perfluorooctane sulfonic acid) and PFOA (perfluorooctanoic acid) being the most studied and understood.

What products contain PFAS?

PFAS have been manufactured and used worldwide since the 1940s and are in many products such as:

- Fire-fighting foam
- Nonstick cookware
- Stain-resistant carpets
- Paints and stains
- Water-resistant fabrics
- Food packaging

Do PFAS cause cancer?

According to the U.S. EPA (Environmental Protection Agency), there is limited evidence that PFAS (PFOS and PFOA) cause cancer in humans.

The International Agency for Research on Cancer (IARC) has classified PFOA as possibly cancer causing.

Correlations between exposure to PFAS and human health effects have been inconsistent.

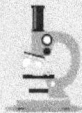

Where can PFAS be found?

PFAS can be found in the environment (air, water, soil) as well as produce products such as vegetables and fruits. PFAS can last a long time in the environment and may be carried over a great distance.

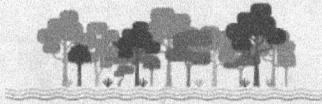

What are the sources of PFAS exposure?

People are most likely exposed by consuming PFAS-contaminated water or food. Exposure may also occur by using products that contain PFAS.

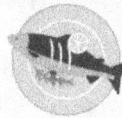

Inhalation and skin exposure are minor exposure pathways. Exposure through skin contact is slow and minor compared to other exposure routes.

Should I get my blood tested for PFAS?

It is not clear how PFAS in blood impacts human health. Having PFAS in your blood does not necessarily mean that you will become ill from PFAS.

A blood test will not provide information for treatment or identify how or where the PFAS exposure occurred. Any decision on testing or treatment should be discussed with your healthcare provider.

PFAS in People

CDC (Centers for Disease Control and Prevention) monitoring estimates that most people in the U.S. will have measurable amounts of PFAS in their blood.

Some PFAS stay in the body for a long time. There is no recommended medical treatment to reduce PFAS in the body.

How can PFAS affect my health?

Effects on health from exposure to low environmental levels of PFAS, such as PFOS and PFOA, are not well known.

Studies in humans and animals are inconclusive.

Findings are limited that exposure leads to increased risk of certain cancers such as prostate, kidney, or testicular cancer.

Non-cancer effects include increased cholesterol levels, impacts on human hormones and the immune system, and fetal and infant developmental effects.

How can I reduce my exposure to PFAS?

You can take the following steps to reduce your risk of exposure:

■Check for fish advisories for water bodies where you fish.

■Follow fish advisories that tell people to stop or limit eating fish from waters contaminated with PFAS or other compounds.

■Read consumer product labels and avoid using products with PFAS.

If your drinking water contains PFAS above the EPA Lifetime Health Advisory, consider using an alternative or treated water source for any activity in which you might swallow water:

■Drinking

■Preparing food

■Cooking

■Brushing teeth

■Preparing infant formula

What are the safe levels of PFAS in Florida's drinking water that do not cause a risk?

The Health Advisory Levels (HALs) for PFOS and PFOA is a combined maximum of 0.07 micrograms per liter (0.07 µg/L) for both.

Contact

If you have questions, please contact the Hazardous Waste Site Health Assessment Team at:

phtoxicology@flhealth.gov

Or call toll free at:

877-798-2772

Learn More

Use the QR code to visit the Florida Department of Health's Hazardous Waste Site Risk Assessment webpage.

Additional information can be found online at:

ATSDR.CDC.gov/pfas

EPA.gov/pfas

www.ingramcontent.com/pod-product-compliance
Lightning Source LLC
Chambersburg PA
CBHW072154270326
41930CB00011B/2421